Confessions
of a
Skinny Girl

How to be Healthy, Happy and Thin
Without Dieting

by

Cecily Rouser

Published by

Balanced Life Publishing Company
Post Office Box 14944
North Palm Beach, Florida 33408
561-625-0250

Credits

Editing by Angela Childers, aschilders1@hotmail.com

Cover photography by Michele Westmorland,
www.Westmorlandphoto.com

IBSN:0-9754002-0-7

Disclaimer

This book is for entertainment purposes only. Every effort has been made to verify the information herein, but no guarantee of correctness is given or implied. Everything in these pages is the writer's opinion, belief or interpretation of events or facts. At no time does the writer state or infer that any information herein is a substitute for advice from qualified professionals.

If the forgoing is unacceptable to you, please return this book to your place of purchase for a full refund.

About the Author

Cecily Rouser has a B.A. in psychology from the University of South Florida and a Masters of Business Administration from Florida Atlantic University. She is a wife and mother, has to get dinner on the table about every night *and* she weighs the same as she did in high school.

Contents

Introduction

Nobody Asks *Me* for Diet Tips

No one ask me for diet tips. It's amazing. People will ask me for advice on almost everything – romance, finance, careers, academics, and wardrobes, even recipes – but nobody ever asks me what I eat on a daily basis. Few people ever ask: "What do you do to stay thin?"

Most skinny people can't tell you what they do anyway. They have natural ways of staying thin that are automatic. It doesn't seem fair, does it?

Then there are those who look great on the outside, but spend their days obsessing about weight control. They can tell you precisely what they do or don't do. If they don't pay attention at all hours of the day, whoops! They pile on another five pounds.

I am sure you've heard that diets don't work. I don't need to rub it in. All the math associated with counting fat grams and calories and carbohydrates and crunches needs to be put to better use.

There are processes, actually *habits,* which anyone can adopt to help them get trim and stay thin without spending every minute worrying about it. The people who have these habits don't even think about them. They just go about their business and don't worry about weight control. These habits work for a lot of us and I'm sure many people are too scared or embarrassed to ask, "What *exactly* are they?"

It's been said that if you do something for 21 days it becomes a habit. But, sometimes the light bulb just goes on and a way to make an immediate change becomes clear. Habits are just something you do every day or frequently. They can be good or bad, but like grains of sand on the beach, they add up to your whole life. Habits can be hard or easy to change. I think it's easy to change a habit if I understand why I want to make the change and how it will benefit me. You probably feel the same way, yet sometimes find it hard to go to the source.

Oh, I've heard people talk amongst themselves in the grocery store and sneak a peak into my cart. I've overheard them say, "I'll bet if we ate like her, we would lose weight." But they *never* say, "Could you show me what you've got in there, please?"

One time a girl asked me what I look for in a plate of food. So I told her. The next time I saw her, she looked terrific. Another time, a girl asked me for some of my (easy) exercises, which I was only too happy to share. The next time I saw her, she looked great, too.

I have my life arranged so that eating well and being active are as easy and enjoyable as possible. My simple approach to food, fun and life works to help me stay healthy and fit. It has worked for my husband and my friends. And I hope it works for you, too.

This book will show you how to handle the subtle, yet constant pressure that has formed us into a nation with little rational sense when it comes to food. It will show you ways to balance activity with food without having to count every calorie and fat gram. It will show you how to set yourself up for success to control weight naturally.

"That Skinny Girl"

I have always been called "that skinny girl." One college roommate even said to a group of friends as we were lying out by the pool, "How would you like to live with that!" while pointing at my body like I should be some kind of outcast. Twenty-five years later, I am 5-foot-six and still weigh 119 pounds.

I gave away my purple hip hugger shorts I wore in high school only because they went out of style. I live my life the way I want to – work hard, play hard and enjoy it all.

The more people I speak with, the more I wonder if I am the only person who made it to adulthood without hang-ups about food. I listen in disbelief to friends and acquaintances discussing their weight control problems and the severe restrictions people put on themselves to prevent weight gain.

People who constantly diet isolate themselves from others. It breaks my heart to hear people say they can't eat this or dine at that restaurant because of their "diet." I have seen people do sit ups between courses to allow themselves the next morsel of food. Even worse are the people who won't let themselves get in the pool or go to the beach or go dancing or get married or anything else until they lose weight.

People will purposely injure their health to control their weight. I formerly managed a ladies clothing store in Boca Raton, Florida. There was a plus-sized women's store close by and I often would chat with the owner about sales. One day, he told me a tale I still have trouble believing.

His wife was a "normal" sized woman, and she often worked in the store. Customers would comment on her size and wonder why she was not a large-sized woman. The owner would say, "She used to be over-weight, but she is very ill and lost a lot of weight due to her illness." Believe it or not, customers would go up and touch her to try to "get" whatever sickness the owner's wife had in an effort to lose weight. Total desperation!

It seems unusual to many that one can eat what she wants and still be happy with her body. I guess I have been lucky. I know it's not that I don't care.

I have had a lot of close experiences with the factors that go into appearance: clothing, make-up and health. My first real job was at a fancy ladies clothing store when I was 16. I worked my way through college behind the cosmetics counter. While in college, I thought I'd like to follow in my mother's footsteps and become a nurse. I took many science and biology courses and studied anatomy and physiology. I loved it, but I was not cut out for nursing school.

My first management job after college was in the clothing industry where I dressed hundreds of women on a weekly basis. I've spoken to thousands of women (and a lot of men, too!) about what it takes to look good.

I've also had exposure to great food and how it can shape lives. My family traveled a lot when I was young and I learned about many different cultures through their food. I still travel as much as possible and always sample the local cuisine.

I love to cook, and cooking and good food have always had an important place in my family. My college roommate could never figure out why I had so many cookbooks. But half of my relatives lived on farms and food was their livelihood. They had the freshest apples from the orchard and corn from next to the lane. The berries came from the berry patch and the eggs were still warm from the chicken.

My grandmothers would bring my sister and me into their kitchens and talk about life while they prepared the family meals. My sister followed in their food-loving footsteps and became a chef. I still have the old Grange cookbook that Grandma gave me when I began to cook.

Please don't assume that because of my metabolism, I can't gain excess weight. I assure you, I can gain plenty. When I went to college for a year in Munich, Germany, I gained the "freshman fifteen" and then some. It might have been twenty pounds, but I didn't have a clue. I still don't know exactly how much weight I had gained because I had *nothing* to gauge my appearance.

I was away from my home for the first time at a college on a military base. It was cold. We lived in old Nazi barracks – the place was gloomy and depressing. I began fixing supper every night for my six-foot-two boyfriend and prepared equal portions for both of us. It was a recipe for weight control disaster.

I also gained fifty pounds when I was pregnant with my daughter. I wasn't happy about the weight gain, but I kept to my habits and lost it all. I even quit smoking after a twelve-year habit, but didn't gain an ounce.

Through sheer luck and circumstance, I have been able to navigate through the landmines of weight control that seem to have tripped up a lot of others. After reflection, I understand how I've managed to maintain a steady, healthy, weight and why techniques many others use don't work. I am happy to share my not-so-secrets with you. There is nothing special to buy. There are no strange techniques to learn. You only have to learn to change your attitude a little. Fortunately, sometimes your attitude is the only thing you *can* change.

My methods are simple and sometimes, easy. After many years of *not* having a weight control problem, I think I have it figured out.

Still, few people take what I have to say seriously when it comes to food. I even have friends who have had lifelong problems with weight control give *me* advice on what to eat. Everybody means well. Everybody has an opinion. And this is mine.

I'm No Movie Star

I am just an everyday person who happens to be happy with her body. You won't see me on the cover of a magazine or on television. You'll see me in line at the grocery or discount store. I'll be at a desk in an office building and in the parent pick up line at school.

Many years ago, a friend of mine said that if I lived in her apartment building, she would be as skinny as me because she would have picked up my habits. So, have a look inside my mind and peer into my cupboards. I'll move in with you for an afternoon. We'll go grocery shopping, take a bike ride around the block and make dinner. I don't buy exotic items at the store. I don't spend my day at the gym. I just use a few simple exercises that I'll share later in the book. Just check with your doctor before trying them. I don't make any claims as to the amount of weight that you'll lose, but my husband read this manuscript and lost 25 pounds soon after. Another friend lost the stubborn 10 pounds she wanted to drop before her wedding.

People can be cruel, regardless of your size. I have had many cruel comments made about me. And I am sure some of us *never* get over the things others say about us. As you read this, you will recognize some of the same people in your life. They may even be you!

Maybe you can take away some of my experiences so you can have the strength to withstand the pressure of others when it comes to food. Maybe this will help people develop their own healthy eating habits. Maybe it also will help parents instill healthy eating habits in their children.

My hope is to help you recondition yourself. I have good memories about eating and still love to eat. I have a friend who says her husband, now deceased, would eat "like he was mad at it." How can you be mad at food? How could this wonderful stuff that does so much for us make a person mad? How awful that he couldn't take pleasure in this life affirming and sustaining act.

My approach to food and life isn't anything fancy. There is nothing to buy that you can't get from a local discount store. Everything I eat comes from neighborhood grocery stores and local restaurants. I don't use any techniques other than common sense and understanding.

All food is energy from the sun. All food begins through the magical process of photosynthesis, which means "made with light." Plants absorb the sun's energy, combine it with chemicals they find in water, air and soil and use it to make the most delicious stuff. The food chain begins with some animals eating plants, other animals eating those animals and humans eating the plant and animal products, too. When we eat too much, the excess energy is stored as fat. Our bodies are like gas tanks – we fill them with fuel and either use the energy or store it. That's it – nothing less and nothing more.

Chapter 1

What Are You Hungry For?

If my "diet" has a name, it is called the "awareness diet." It's not the "obsessive diet." With my busy life, I don't have time to weigh myself constantly or count calories. I can't spend a lot of time preparing special meals and shopping in many different stores. I don't even know anybody who lives such a luxurious life. I am simply aware of why I eat, what I eat and where my food comes from.

Many exercise and lifestyle disciplines focus on the mind-body connection. These are great. It is so easy to become disconnected from your feelings, your motivations and your actions, and it often takes a conscious effort to get back in touch with them.

We are pulled in so many directions at once, have so many demands placed on us, that sometimes we are so out of balance that we sleepwalk through life. We don't have time to think about how we really feel, and lose touch with the simple things that make life worth living.

I read an article once about a couple struggling to save their marriage. The counselor had asked the wife repeatedly what she needed for herself. The couple had been to many sessions before the wife finally blurted out: "I want to take a bubble bath."

That was it! A little pampering, a little solitude, a little time to think were what she needed most. She had been so intent on pleasing others that she had placed her simplest need on hold. Does this sound familiar? I am sure the couple had many other issues to deal with, but it's a story that illustrates how easy it is to get out of sync, and the importance of a balanced life.

I am convinced that having a life out of balance is a main contributor to overeating. So many people eat to fill a void. But can that void be filled with food? Is it really food that is needed?

My food satisfies my hunger for food. That's all. I don't use food as a substitute to satisfy my hunger for anything else. If you really want something, don't reach for the refrigerator if you're hungry for something other than food.

I believe most cravings should be explored, rather than denied. Try to figure out what *you* really want. People hunger for love, companionship, solitude, success, recognition, attention, appreciation, beauty, relaxation, excitement and hundreds of other things that are so personal, I wouldn't want to try to list them. If you feel a void, the void is there, the void is real. Fill it with something other than food. Take action to fill your needs — satisfy what you are craving. It isn't always food.

Sometimes we deny, even to ourselves, that what we need is real. Or we deny our needs because we feel we don't deserve to satisfy them. Denial is an experience shared by everyone who has ever suffered a loss. Of the "Seven Stages of Grief" described by Dr. Elizabeth Kubler-Ross in her groundbreaking book, *On Death and Dying,* denial is the very first. She, of course, was referring to the grieving process associated with the death of a loved one. But I have seen people, including myself, in denial about every human experience imaginable. For years, I was even in denial about the breed of my dog.

I listened to a woman on TV trying to explain her severe weight gain. She said that one day she "just woke up" and weighed 400 pounds! How can you "just wake up" one day and be 400 pounds? The day before that she must have weighed 399 pounds. She had to have been in serious denial of everything in life to "just wake up" and find herself in that predicament.

Sometimes it is so hard to acknowledge that what you want IS what you want. People rationalize: "If I deny this hunger, or fill it in another way, I won't have to face it." I think this is the biggest hurdle people must overcome when fighting a weight problem. It isn't knowledge or willpower. Overweight people are filled with wisdom and strength. I've heard it said that, when fighting a weight problem, it's not what you *eat*, but what's eating *you*. It's also learning when you are hungry, learning when you are full and listening to the hunger cues and what they are really telling you.

When I was first dating my husband, he commented about the amount of food I had left on my plate. As a member of the "Clean-Plater Club," he thought I should eat more. I looked him in the eye and said, "I eat when I'm hungry and stop when I'm full. Is that so unusual?" He got quiet for a moment, and said, "Yes, it is."

I *only* eat when I'm hungry. I don't eat for any other reason, except once in a while for taste. I'll even say out loud, "I'm only eating this because it tastes *sooo* good."

So, feel what you're feeling. Is it real hunger or not? I know someone who said she doesn't know what it feels like to be hungry. She says she always eats before she's hungry.

I don't believe in deprivation for anyone, but it makes no sense to me to eat when you're not hungry. Hunger for food feels like a gnawing in the stomach. You can hear growls and gurgling noises. If it is too far past mealtime for me, I start to feel a little light-headed and I get really grouchy. If my family and I are in the car and I start complaining about everything, my husband heads straight for the nearest drive through to get me something to eat.

I am aware of my hunger, and what I need to satisfy that hunger. In later chapters, I will discuss ways that I fill my hunger for food and my hunger for other things as well. Fortunately, a lot of my "fillers" can help keep pounds off, too.

It's not only awareness, however, that contributes to my "non-diet" success. It's just the little things that I do, my habits, and my life, that keep me "a skinny girl."

To get you thinking about positive changes, fill in the following blanks:

A. I am hungry for: _____

B: I want to: _____

C: I will do it on: circle one

Monday   Tuesday   Wednesday   Thursday

Friday   Saturday   Sunday

D: I will do it again on: circle one more

Monday   Tuesday   Wednesday   Thursday

Friday   Saturday   Sunday

Chapter 2

Ban the Clean-Plater Club!

Everybody knows the Clean-Plater Club. It's when somebody (usually a big person) tells somebody else (usually a little person) that they need to eat all the food on their plate or they won't get dessert or some equally disastrous consequence.

I firmly believe that the Clean-Plater Club causes people to ignore their normal "full" response and conditions them to overeat three or more times a day. The normal satiation response becomes so weak that it ceases to function.

I know people who eat until the food is gone, with no exceptions. No matter how much there is, they will eat until the food is gone. They can spend hours at a buffet and do nothing but fill plate after delicious plate and clean them all.

The first time I made dinner for my now-husband, I made one of my favorite dishes, beef stroganoff. I served him a nice portion and he ate it all. Seeing that he had "cleaned his plate," I gave him another serving. He ate it all. Seeing that he had "cleaned his plate," I got ready to give him another serving. When he saw me heading toward him with the serving spoon in my hand, he finally said, "Whoa! No more! I can't eat another bite!" I said, "But you ate everything on your plate." And his response was, "But I'm supposed to."

To me, eating everything on your plate means that you are still hungry. If you stop eating when you are full, you will always leave something on your plate. It will happen *every* time. There is *no way* to gauge, just by looking, how much of a particular food you need and to measure it out precisely.

Many people can't stand this concept. I can't tell you the number of people who have tried to make me eat everything on my plate, whether I wanted to or not. If this is you – STOP IT!

Getting fat will not help the children starving in India or China or anywhere else. Someone once said to me, in anger, that if I sent my leftovers to India, the people there would eat it, no matter how rotten. This person had never been to India: How would he know? The main issue in this disagreement was control. He had no interest in helping anybody and was only trying to make me feel bad. If this is something that you do to yourself or to other people – STOP IT RIGHT NOW!

Parents are always doing this to children. I cringe every time I overhear parents say, "Eat everything on your plate," to their child. The child then overeats to please the parent or mealtimes become a battleground. Either way, the child loses.

I think one of the reasons I have sane eating habits is because my parents *never once* told me to clean my plate or forced me to eat anything I didn't want. I was always served small portions with the assurance that if I ate that, I was welcome to "seconds." Sometimes I asked, but most times I didn't. And I never went hungry.

Today, I will usually say to my family and guests, "If you eat all that, I will give you more." I always keep something in reserve. If people want seconds, they are there for the taking. If they don't, we have leftovers for another meal. I also save desserts for at least a half hour after the meal, if I serve them at all, so the issue of saving room for dessert doesn't come up. Between meals and dessert, we clean the kitchen or go for a walk. By waiting a bit, the full feeling sinks in and the urge for sweets diminishes or even goes away.

I apply the same "If you eat all that, I will give you more" rule to treats as well. Nobody craves these things because they are there for the taking – right at eye level – not hidden or forbidden. The strange thing is: I often have to throw out baked goods because they have become stale and I toss out the Halloween candy around Christmas.

Do not eat because people are starving anywhere. It will not help anybody if you or someone you love gets fat. If you are worried about people who are starving, do something real for them. There are people without enough to eat in your own neighborhood. If you feel guilty about throwing food away, let that guilt motivate you to help out someone less fortunate than yourself.

Listen to your body when it tells you that you are full. Try to make your internal controls work again. Your internal control may be a small, tiny voice inside you saying, "No thank you. Really, I've had all I want." It may be so faint you hardly hear it, but listen to *it*, not anybody else.

My internal control says, "Put the fork down and step away from the table, please." I listen every time.

The Business of Eating

When you're out to eat, don't be afraid to eat your fill and take the rest "to go." I've had servers look at me with distain when I've ordered a "doggy bag," as if I was insulting the chef for not eating it all. The server is there to serve *you*, not the other way around. What you do with the leftovers is *your* business.

And restaurants *are* businesses. The managers are trained to get a certain amount of money out of each table per hour that the business is open. When the quota is not being met, the managers have a choice: "turn over" more tables or raise prices.

We've all been to those restaurants where you look *up* to order. The garish orange décor is designed to get you out of there fast. It is so uncomfortable that the turnover is automatic. Most people would rather just "drive-through" and not even stop in.

At restaurants where you look *down* to order, they often cannot turn over tables by rushing you out, so they raise the prices. To retain customers, they give more food for the money. Because food costs are often a small portion of overhead (what it costs to run the place), the increase in prices is profitable.

The real problem is: What do *you* do when you're faced with more food? Do your internal controls work? Internal controls don't work for a lot of people. They've ignored them for so long that they don't even notice them anymore.

If you've forgotten what feeling full is like, use external controls. It may be a pair of pants that feel just a little too tight when you're sitting down. When you get that feeling, pay attention and stop eating. Forget the Clean-Plater Club. Tear up your membership card. Don't recruit others, either.

If you can't train yourself to leave food on your plate, *don't supersize it*! Don't supersize anything! Servers are trained to ask you if you want to supersize it. Oh, it's only 39 cents; don't you always say, "Yes?" You have to practice saying, "No. Thank you." even if you have to do it in front of a mirror. Usually, you're just saying no to a speaker box anyway. There *is* a person behind it, but I promise these workers won't take it personally. I always order medium; it's a habit.

At restaurants, you can order an appetizer instead of an entrée. Really. They will allow you to do that. I often order an appetizer and a salad – if it's what I want. I think they are on to me, though, because appetizer portions seem to be growing, too. You can even split portions with someone else. Sometimes there is a "sharing charge," but I'd rather pay extra than waddle o ut.

You *don't* have to order it all, and then eat it all. If you've been conditioned to eat it all, do everything you can to recondition yourself. Make a conscious effort to understand your own feelings, and then pay attention to them. I guarantee it's worth it. *You* are worth it.

Chapter 3

Required Equipment For A Skinny Girl

If you come to my house, you will see certain things I can't live my life without. First and foremost is my attitude: I look at food very differently than most people.

I *never* look at food as "fattening" or "non -fattening." I never feel I've been "bad" when I eat certain things. Every food has a place in my "non-diet." I look at foods as "rich" or "filling." To me, a piece of cake is "rich," not fattening or forbidd en.

Very often, I will say to myself that I need to eat *more* of something that will do me good, never less. I have never said that I need to eat less of this or that, but that I need to eat more apples, for example.

I practice healthy selfishness. My attitude toward food is "What are you doing *for* me?" I don't think of it in terms of what food is doing "to" me. I never look at a particular food and believe that it will go to a specific place on my body, such as my hips or arms. I want to know: Is my food giving me strong bones and teeth and glossy hair? Does it have proteins and carbohydrates, vitamins and minerals? Is it giving me the energy to get out of bed in the morning and take on my day? Does it taste good? If the answer to these questions is "no," I look for something else.

The answers to nutrition questions are so easy to find. Nutrition information is on everything these days. By law, it is printed on all processed foods. Many stores offer nutritional information on non-processed foods as well. Even restaurants are listing nutritional information for the dishes they serve. The information label even tells you what percentage of a certain nutrient you are getting for your money. Sometimes, it's none at all. You don't need a calculator, but pay attention if there are too many zeros in the nutrient column and not enough zeros in the fats column.

In order to be aware of what you eat and what it is doing for you, you must have the equipment to set yourself up for success. With these items and activities, I find that success with weight control is automatic. You won't be able to fool yourself into thinking you know what you're doing when you really don't. The truth can hurt, but it can set you free.

The Skinny Girl's Bathroom

There are a few essentials I can't live without in my bathroom. The first is least one:

Full-Length Mirror

Have you ever heard the old adage, "You can never be too rich or too thin?" It wasn't about the béarnaise sauce. The now famous saying coined by the early 20th century Duchess of Windsor has been quoted by people around the world. Could we consider the source of this "wisdom?" As anyone with any common sense knows, it is quite possible for people to be too rich, and quite possible for people to be too thin.

I believe that the Duchess was known for nothing but her outward appearance and social climbing skills. I would be happy to find out if she had contributed anything to our society other than her fantastic posture and this ridiculously overrated phrase. As far as I know, she and her (third) husband spent most of their time as guests of other (rich) people.

Please, let's not use this woman as an example of a fulfilling life for the rest of us. Being rich or thin or both does not make one a better person. It's what you do for others, especially those who can't "pay back," that makes one a better person.

I am bringing this up because there *is* one thing that the rich and the thin have in common. That one thing is a mirror. Lots and lots of mirrors.

The Hall of Mirrors at Versailles is only one example. Built by King Louis XIV of France, Versailles is a testament to opulence. The Hall of Mirrors is its most famous feature. The room seems to extend for a mile. Mirrors are used to make the already enormous space seem even larger.

Most fabulous homes have great walls of mirrors in the foyer, in the dining room and especially in the bath and dressing rooms.

At fancy department stores, dressing rooms have mirrors angled on two or more walls. These huge rooms also have modeling platforms and shoes of different heel heights to provide customers with the best idea of how they'll look in their new clothes.

In dance studios and exercise gyms (places noted for people who are in shape), mirrors line every wall.

It is quite a change, however, when moving from the rich to the poor, or upscale to the affordable. In discount stores, clothes are tried on in a tiny room with *no mirrors.* In rental apartments, "starter homes" and dorm rooms, the only mirror hangs above the bathroom sink. Because the view is only from the neck up, it's like the rest of the body doesn't exist.

It is in these cheap places where most of us set up house for the first time and forge our own eating habits. If we have little or no feedback as to how we are doing, we can develop some pretty unhealthy habits.

Before placing decorative mirrors around your house, get yourself a full-length mirror. A skinny girl must own a full-length mirror, preferably two. You can get them at the discount store for less than $12.

One should be placed where you can regularly see a clear view of yourself without any clothes. Only then will you get an idea of your true size and what you need and want to accomplish. One of two things will happen. Either you will *not* like what you see and lose your appetite, or you *will* like what you see and think, "Not too shabby!" Either way, you win!

If you have two mirrors, they should be set up facing each other at an angle so you can get a view of yourself from *all* sides.

Am I advocating that we become a nation of narcissists? Not at all. Whether it is fair or not, we are judged by our appearance. Unconsciously, people will decide if you deserve their attention within the first seven seconds of meeting you – and that's if you're lucky. If you are not lucky, you will have even less time to make a good impression.

Humans, as a species, usually decide instantly as to what kind of relationship they want with others based on their looks. If people present themselves as worthwhile and important, they will be treated accordingly. The opposite is also true.

You need to see a 360-degree view of yourself before leaving the house. This means standing in front of a mirror and looking at yourself from all sides. It takes time to dress *and* assess, but it also takes time to obsess over extra pounds.

Take the time to look good. You deserve it and it pays off 100 times over in the feedback you receive from others. When you know you look good, it shows through to other people. They pay attention to you and really listen to what you have to say. People treat me much better when I look good and when I *know* I look good.

This last look in the mirror is not vanity. It is preparing you to meet the world and its challenges. It is setting you up for positive feedback and success. If you are successful at your endeavors, then you can pass your blessings onto others. I find I can be much more generous to others with my time and money when I am successful than when I am struggling to make ends meet. And if what goes around *really* comes around, then the cycle can start all over again.

If you can't stomach the idea of a full-length mirror in the bathroom, just get one for the back of the bedroom door. Then move it to the bathroom after you've become comfortable with the idea of having it there.

Bathroom Scale

You need access to a scale to see how much you really weigh. Yes, you really have to look. The one at the grocery store will do. The one at the gym is fine. Or you can even buy one. I don't advocate stepping on a scale every day. Weighing yourself once a week is plenty, and once a month is fine if you are happy with your weight. If you see the numbers creeping up, you are storing too much energy. Then you have three choices: eat less, eat differently or raise your activity level. This book has hundreds of different ways to help you succeed in your choice. Although some may disagree, you simply need to have an idea of how much you weigh. If you're not happy with it – take some action! Being aware of your weight is the start.

Massager or Loofah Sponge for the Tub

A massager is a wonderful indulgence that provides a lot of benefit for a little time and money. A loofah sponge is a natural gourd that expands when wet. They cost about $2 at discount stores. Massagers are made of plastic and rubber, have little nubs on the massaging surface and slip over your hand. The pricier massagers have a space for a fancy bar of "anti-cellulite" soap and can be found at department stores.

Soap up a loofah or massager and rub it all over the next time you are in the shower or tub. The effect of each is the same: it gets the circulation going in your skin – your largest organ. Massagers exfoliate your body like a masque exfoliates your face. The result is smooth and glowing skin. I don't believe people need supplements to "rid the body of toxins." The stimulation of a loofah or massager enhances the cleansing action that your circulation system already has in place.

Fitness Equipment

I *have* to have a bicycle. I use my bicycle at least twice a week to take a ride around the block. Even five minutes is a mini-vacation. It is better for relieving stress than a box of donuts anytime. My family and I like to take rides together in the evening and just enjoy each other's company. The fresh air and wind in your hair can really clear your head. Pedaling makes your blood move oxygen to every cell in your body, raising your metabolism. It's great for your heart and doesn't pollute the atmosphere. What more could you ask for?

We have great bike paths in our town, but they have been a rather new addition. If you enjoy biking but don't have decent places to ride, write your state representatives on the transportation committee. Their addresses are in the phone book. They decide which projects, like bike paths and heart trails, are funded with your tax dollars. They work for you and they'll listen.

If you don't want to bike, what else do you like to do outside? Get comfortable in a sporting goods store. Just look around. You don't have to buy anything. Look at all the equipment options available to get you up and moving.

Spend time studying the equipment. You'll likely find something that you like to do. My local sporting goods store has everything from fishing equipment to jump ropes.

If you've forgotten how to use the equipment or have never seen an inline skate, find a kid to teach you how to use the equipment and go along for the ride. There's a double bonus! You get ideas and motivation to exercise and the child receives some individual respect and attention.

Winter weather may prevent you from biking or whatever you choose to do outdoors. There are many other activities to get you out of the house and help clear your mind. The stationary bikes at a gym are a good substitute, but get the real thing and use it, if you can. If you're in a cold weather climate, try ice-skating, cross-country skiing, or snowshoeing. Enjoy the invigorating air. You don't need to go to a gym to be fit.

Roman Chair

This may be the best invention since the bicycle. I have been using a Roman chair for "reverse sit-ups" for over 30 years. A "reverse sit-up" is just like it sounds. Rather than lying on your back, you lie on your stomach. Then you arch your back and lift your torso up from the floor.

Many gyms have Roman chairs, but I finally bought one for my home. It has two supports coming up from the ground, a padded bar for your stomach on one support and a bar to hook your legs under on the other support. You drape yourself over the stomach support with your head hanging down, hook your legs under the leg bar and lift yourself parallel to the ground.

There is *nothing* better than a Roman chair for exercising and strengthening *all* of the back muscles from your neck to your ankles at one time. There is *nothing* in daily life that even approximates this movement. And there is *nothing* that provides so much benefit in such a short period of time. Just four or five "reverse sit-ups," two or three times a week, take less than 30 seconds and really get the kinks out. Having your back muscles in shape prevents back problems and gives you great posture. Also, anything you do to strengthen your back will strengthen your stomach muscles as well.

If I don't have access to a Roman chair, I just hook my feet under a piece of heavy furniture and lift my torso off the floor.

These simple things: a mirror, a scale, a loofah and some simple exercise machines form the basis of my "skinny life."

Now, on to the kitchen:

A Skinny Girl's Kitchen

We are going to go through every drawer and cupboard in <u>Chapter 12</u>. I will tell you what I have and where it is stored and why, but these are my absolute essentials.

Water

A major component of livin' skinny is a ready supply of fresh, cold water to drink. It helps if you have it filtered, too. The health benefits of filtered and bottled water versus tap water are debatable, but I find that filtered water just tastes better.

Store your water so it is the easiest beverage to reach. The "cold water in the door" refrigerators are terrific. If you don't have the refrigerator option, stock your fridge with bottled water or always keep a jug of filtered water available.

I don't measure out eight glasses (64 ounces) of water a day like some diets recommend. How would you get out of the house? I think "eight glasses" is a benchmark for total water intake from all sources. There is plenty of water in most foods that you eat and beverages that you drink.

Dehydration is a real problem for many of us. It can cause nasty headaches and a host of other health problems. Many people mistake thirst for hunger pangs and eat instead of drinking water. That's really a big mistake, too.

I stay away from carbonated beverages as my everyday drinks. Years ago, I would buy soda by the case – that made it the easiest beverage to reach for when I was thirsty. I still drink a soda now and then, but, besides water, I usually choose milk, fruit or vegetable juices if I want some flavor. Some juices (like orange juice) are too rich for me, so I mix them with water, club soda or ginger ale for an afternoon "cocktail."

If you look at the nutrition labels on fruit juices, they are loaded with good things for you. There is not a single thing in a can of soda that will help you look or feel good. A person can only go without water for a day or two without suffering severe or fatal health problems. Read the label on a soda can: you can go a *lifetime* without *any* of those ingredients.

Fat Gram Counter

You don't need to buy a fat gram counter book or memorize the fat and calories of everything you eat. But borrow one for an afternoon and spend some time getting to know the fat content of the foods you eat. It's all listed there in black and white. Some of these counters will tell you to limit your fat intake to 22 grams of fat per day. I agree that it is wise to limit your fat intake, but that is ridiculous. I couldn't do that for more than a day. Fat is where the flavor is!

When I looked at the fat content of what I was eating and compared it to my activity level, I decided 50 grams of fat a day was a good amount for me. You will have to decide an amount that is healthy and works best for you. In Chapter 11, I'll discuss my choices when it comes to fats and what they do *for* me and not *to* me.

The fat gram counter can help you find out where your fat is coming from. Then *you* decide if that's the source you want to receive it from each day. I found I was getting 50 grams of fat *just from my morning coffee*. I needed to make a change or I was heading for trouble.

The fat gram counter is important because of "food jags." Everyone has "food jags." It's when you eat the same thing for breakfast two weeks in a row. Or when you buy the same lunch every day for a week or a month. Or eat the same snacks at the movies. Even the editor of *Martha Stewart Living* magazine will admit to eating the same thing every morning. And they probably have test kitchens right in the office!

Anyone who has ever worked in a restaurant will tell you most people order the same thing over and over. I do it all the time. I settle on my favorite dish in my favorite restaurant and hate to change.

This is because we only live on about ten types of food. We may eat different versions of the same thing, but really, most people live on ten items that are the staple foods of their lives. Think about it. What *are* your staple foods?

Take a hard look at what is in your kitchen and on your grocery list right now. These are your "usual food choices," your ten staple foods. You have them. Be critical and find out what they are and if they are helping you. If not, change them to foods that will do good things *for* you, not bad things *to* you. My list is in <u>Chapter 10</u>.

One afternoon, take two hours to measure the amount of fat in your staple foods. How much fat is in your serving of coffee cream? What is in the mayonnaise you spread on a typical sandwich? What do you put in your chicken salad? Don't forget the butter you put on potatoes or the dressings you use on salads. The drive-through burger you get every day counts, too.

Line them all up and measure them out. Add it up. If you're going over your total – cut back! Make some changes. I don't mean buying fat free, tasteless alternatives, but if a choice is there, make sure it's the best choice for *you*.

Every diet needs a little fat to be healthy. I don't eat a lot of fat, but as I said before, fat is where the flavor is. One change I made was to substitute regular milk for my coffee cream instead of half and half. Over months and years, every little bit helps.

Food Scale

Recently, I broke down and bought a food scale. I use it to divide up mega packs of food, such as ground beef, into manageable portions to freeze for later use. I also bought it so I could find out how a USDA serving size from the "food pyramid" was *supposed* to look. It's a lot smaller than we think, and the portion recommendations definitely don't correlate with the serving sizes used by manufacturers or restaurants. There is no "American" or "Metric" standard serving size. Although I might measure out ingredients when I cook a dish, I surely don't measure food when I am scrambling to get dinner on the table.

Take an afternoon and measure out a serving size of your staple foods. What you think is a serving size may be completely different from what the scale reveals.

Read the nutrition information to see if your usual choices are providing the necessary nutrition you need. This is what nutritionists mean when they say to "read labels." If you're not getting enough of some nutrient or getting too much of another, make some changes. I did when I began having trouble maintaining my energy throughout the day and had an insatiable craving for salt.

I discovered I wasn't getting enough potassium from either my usual food choices or my multi-vitamins. I substituted a salt and potassium mixture (found in the seasonings aisle in the grocery store) for my regular table salt at home. It made a big difference in my energy level – *and* my potato chip consumption! I often add foods to my diet that will keep me healthy. Sometimes they aren't my first food choices, but since they are "good for me" and I enjoy most foods, I add a serving. Sometimes two bites is a large enough serving size for me.

Vegetable Steamer, Cutting Board and Good Knife

When I worked as a make-up artist for several national brands, I couldn't resist asking the women with good skin what they ate on a regular basis. Nine times out of ten, vegetables were at the top of their lists.

It may sound boring, but vegetables, grains and beans, in all their glorious colors, are the basis of what I eat. I usually start with them when planning my meals. These aren't just in salads, but I enjoy them in all different forms, from steamed to stir fried to soups.

I certainly enjoy a steak now and then. I'm not a vegetarian by any stretch of the imagination, but I usually use meat and other animal products as side dishes – not the main event. I'll share some recipes with you later, so you'll understand how vegetables can be the stars of the show. And everyone needs to eat *more* of those!

It is important to be careful when preparing vegetables. We've all seen those overcooked, soggy messes that have passed for vegetables on some relative's dinner table. Don't cook them like that! It's no wonder people don't like to eat their vegetables.

Spinach, for instance, is wonderful at breakfast, lunch or dinner. Most people only remember the overcooked and limp version they were served in childhood. Fortunately for me, my dad hated spinach, so I only started eating it when I was old enough to appreciate it in Greek and French cuisine. What a difference!

Skinny people eat their vegetables. However, to properly prepare them, you need the proper tools.

I have a little microwave vegetable steamer that is nothing fancy at all. It might have cost $5, if that much. Just put in cut up vegetables, add a cup of water or broth and microwave on high for five to eight minutes, depending on the vegetable's density, add a little flavoring like garlic, spray margarine or soy sauce and you're done. It's a great timesaver when putting meals together at the last minute.

A skinny person also has a big cutting board. I gave up on fancy wooden ones. They are way too hard to take care of and harbor germs. I like those big, white plastic cutting boards that fit in the dishwasher. Mine is used almost every time I cook a meal. I own boards in several sizes and some days I use all of them. I bought a multi-pack of cutting boards at my local warehouse store for about $12.

Another kitchen necessity for a skinny girl is a good quality knife. It's a big investment, but they last a lifetime. The knife can't come from a discount store. It needs to be heavy, with the "tang" running all the way through the handle. It must be stainless steel, so it won't warp or rust. Mine cost well over $100 and *that* was on sale, but my knife has been a terrific investment. It has made my life easier. It slices through everything with little effort on my part and actually makes chopping fun and therapeutic.

Wok

I love my wok. It's the main tool used to prepare the Eastern diet, which is so healthy. Mine is electric, so I can cook with it anywhere. It goes in the dishwasher, so it's easy to take care of. I try to use it once a week.

With a wok, you can prepare fantastic tasting vegetables, seafood and lean meats in just a bit of oil. The food is cooked quickly, so it retains all of its great flavor. And you can find fantastic ways to use up leftovers from other meals.

I sometimes kid people that Mexican food is all the same items cooked in different ways, and that Chinese food is all different items cooked in the same way. That's not really true, of course, but Eastern cuisine features so many different vegetables and meats, cut into small pieces, and cooked quickly. The taste and nutrients stay intact.

Some people say they don't like Chinese food or believe it's "bad" for you. I think most of these people have only eaten Chinese food out of a can (another soggy mess) and have heard too much bad press about MSG.

MSG is the chemical abbreviation for a very popular flavor enhancer probably sitting in your cupboard right now. It "wakes up flavor" by causing a chemical reaction on your tongue, making your taste buds more receptive. Is this bad? I don't know. I do know that I can feel it instantly when too much MSG is in my meal. My face starts to twitch and feels tight. Fortunately, I haven't had that sensation in many years, probably because people are more aware of what they put into food. Either way, I prefer to enhance the flavors of my foods by cooking them right rather than adding chemical enhancements.

Vitamins

Everyone needs tiny quantities of certain nutrients to live. Ask anyone who has had a thyroid problem how important it is to have everything in balance. It's impossible for anyone to measure out and eat precise quantities of what our bodies need. I hedge my bets with vitamins.

I am sure that in centuries past, people's activity levels were high enough to merit eating substantial quantities of unprocessed foods – foods with their vitamins intact. More people lived and worked on farms and weight control was not the issue it is today.

Someone once told me, "We don't need vitamins because we eat!" Well, of course we eat, but what do we eat? Most of us cannot possibly eat as much as our forebears could to get the nutrients we need.

I don't believe we should be taking huge doses of vitamins, which can cause serious health problems, but I know my energy level slips if I haven't had my multi-vitamin. Years ago, I spent some time in the drugstore looking at all the vitamin choices. There are hundreds. I decided on a multi-vitamin with extra iron. But even my careful choice does not give me all of the nutrients I need, so I look to other sources of potassium, phosphorus, magnesium and calcium. Chapter 10 and the Appendix contain a list of foods that can help you get necessary vitamins and minerals into your diet. If your multi-vitamin doesn't have everything you need, you can make a *conscious* effort to add foods that do.

Now you've had a glimpse into some of my household cabinets, and have seen the items I must have to maintain balance in my life. I'll share more about them in upcoming chapters.

Chapter 4

Your Body Isn't Stupid

I never think of my body as a traitor. It's a tool for fulfilling my goals and ambitions. It doesn't define who I am – it helps me do what I want to do. I have to take good care of it. I appreciate it and treat it as well as I can.

Your body is a miracle of chemistry and engineering. You have 300 trillion cells serviced by 12,000 miles of blood vessels. They all have important work to do.

We do all kinds of stupid things to our bodies and they deal as best as they can. We cut ourselves and our circulation systems send white blood cells and platelets to clot the blood and seal the wound. We go out in bright sunlight and our eyes squint so they won't be damaged. We get off-balance and our arms (usually) catch us before we fall.

Everything you do, everything you see, every thought you have is an electrical or chemical reaction. These reactions happen instantaneously, so you feel pain when you cut yourself, blink when the light is too bright, and put your arms out when you fall.

The nerves in your body form a network that reach from your brain to each and every cell. They are encased in a protective substance called myelin that is made of fat. Each nerve must have this protective coating to ensure that messages reach the right destination.

Each nerve sends messages from one end to the other by electricity. The nerves have little spaces between them called synapses. A chemical from one nerve washes across the space to causes a reaction in the next nerve. Then, another chemical washes over the space to stop the reaction. This is how we move a muscle or see a sunset. Real problems occur when the body lacks the nutrients to produce these chemicals or when damage occurs to the myelin coating on the nerves.

So, why do we *really* eat? The biological basis is to sustain these electro-chemical reactions. The other reason is to make life fun and interesting.

Think about it. The pleasure you receive from an activity is usually tied directly with the food involved. Picnics, boating, entertaining, vacations, luncheons, brunches, and business meetings: all have a food component. Business deals are made over a steak dinner. Engagements are formed over a fancy meal. Food is interwoven with everything we do for enjoyment. It is no wonder that people associate food with good feelings.

With all of these food-related activities to deal with every day, how do you distinguish between what you want and what you really need? Hunger is your body's way of telling you something. Wanting is a type of hunger, and if it gets you what you really need, then hunger is good. But, don't eat food if you are hungry for something else. Listen and make sure the right message is getting through. Your body doesn't want to be fat. Look at all the ways it objects to extra weight. Excess weight affects every single metabolic process in your body and can ultimately lead to premature death. Do you think your body wants that?

It is so important to be in touch with what your body needs. I find I crave what is good for me. Sometimes it's tough to make a distinction as to what I really crave – like potassium. But, it pays to investigate cravings, not ignore them.

I am happier today with my body than I was in my twenties. That may seem unlikely, but I am happier with myself, and my body was a critical part of that journey. I have never asked anyone if "this makes me look fat." I am proud of the pouf of my stomach because I grew my child in there.

There's another part of my body that I appreciate. And many women spend hundreds of dollars to remove it. You probably won't believe this, but I *really*, actually *appreciate* my cellulite. Here is why.

Anyone who *doesn't* have cellulite was born a man. Men don't *need* it. Cellulite is what keeps a woman's butt from crashing down around her ankles when she's pregnant. It is *supposed* to be there. It is "caused" by a *normal* crisscross pattern in the structure under the skin of the leg: a *normal* woman's leg.

Think about it. What else has a crisscross pattern? Nets! Fishnets, hairnets, acrobatic nets – all made for strength and to keep objects from falling. When a woman is pregnant, her body endures tremendous pressure. In addition to myriad other changes, her blood volume doubles to support the new life. This process would wreak havoc on a body that had no cellulite. Anyone who has experienced extreme swelling can attest to the damage it inflicts on tissues. It is *not* caused by certain kinds of fat or by toxins – it's just there. It can even be seen under the skin of babies, and they don't *have* toxins in them. All the so-called cures are only offered to separate you from your money. If you have cellulite, it is because you are a woman and what is wrong with that?

When I managed a clothing store, women trying on swimsuits would get so upset because of their cellulite. We would tell them, "Just tan it and forget it. People look at your face, not your butt." With what we know about sun exposure today, I would say, "Get out the sunless tanner," but I would still tell them to forget it. The massager in the shower will get your circulation going so your skin is healthier and more taut, but I still value my cellulite as a part of who I am. And if you have cellulite or love someone who does – I think you should learn to value it, too.

I once read that diets don't work because when a person grows a fat cell, they can never lose it. The theory is that it's there in the body forever and dieting will cause it to shrink, but it will never go away. I think each cell in your body has a life span – it is created, lives for a time, dies and is sloughed off with other dead cells. Your skin loses cells constantly. Your hair is a long strand of dead cells. Some people think that fat cells don't work that way. Personally, I think that would mean a fat cell is immortal, like a cancer cell. Either way, I don't think of fat cells as being cardboard boxes that take up space, but rather as plastic sandwich bags or balloons. When they are empty, they take up practically no space at all.

Because fat is stored energy, your body will draw on it when it needs a source for fuel, just like it will draw on a mother's teeth if she doesn't have enough calcium to grow bones for her baby. But when you eat too much, your fat cells will expand, balloon, and store the excess energy. Just like cells of a hibernating animal, your fat cells assume you will need that energy for a purpose, and will store and store until the day you burn it off.

Smoking is Stupid

I wish I had listened to my body the first time I tried a cigarette. I coughed, I felt sick to my stomach. I got a headache. My body tried to let me know I was making a mistake. But, I didn't listen. I smoked the second cigarette and got hooked. I will never be that stupid again! Smoking is an addiction for most people, and those who say they can quit at any time are wrong. I think some sort of switch in the brain flips during that second cigarette to make the whole body crave nicotine.

I quit smoking after 12 years and didn't gain an ounce. It was the hardest and best decision I've ever made.

I have spoken to people who refuse to quit smoking for fear of gaining weight. Quitting smoking without gaining weight can be done! I did it. Cancer is a sure method of losing weight, but most of us would rather enjoy the victory standing up, not lying in a hospital bed. I choose other options to stay thin.

When a person smokes, damage is not only done to the lungs. All of the body's processes are affected. The smoke in the lungs replaces the vital oxygen that enables each cell in the body to function. Rather, the oxygen is replaced by nasty, harmful chemicals.

With less oxygen, the skin loses its tautness. As a makeup artist, I could identify a smoker from five feet away. A smoker's skin is in horrible shape. It doesn't receive what it needs to replace its cells properly. After years of addiction, skin looks poisoned. It takes on a yellowish cast and looks as if it has eroded.

Similar damage occurs to the eyes. Eyesight degeneration is common in long-term smokers. The list of the harmful effects of smoking is endless. I could go on and on. There is nothing positive about smoking. It's not a habit – it's an addiction.

Many people have paired alcohol consumption with nicotine consumption. They say they can't have a drink without a cigarette, so they believe they must quit drinking (and end their social life) if they quit smoking.

That is simply not true. Many people give up cigarettes without having to sacrifice their social lives. If you are holding on to smoking as a means of staying thin, or are just afraid to quit, here's how I quit without gaining weight.

Recognize that there are two stages to quitting smoking

First, there is the social basis of smoking, which is why everyone starts in the first place. No one would ever start if a "friend" didn't give him or her that first cigarette. People use smoking as a basis of conversation and connecting with others. Asking another person for a cigarette or a light used to be an acceptable way of beginning conversations with interesting-looking people. Asking a buddy if he wanted to go outside for a smoke was another way to connect. You got a break and a few minutes to talk.

Now, consider alternatives for going out with a buddy for a cigarette. Invite friends to join you for a walk or a short bike ride, or to have a cold drink – anything but a smoke. There is no need to give up the social aspects of smoking. Just spend some time thinking of good substitutes.

The social aspect of smoking also includes the physical habit of lighting up. That hand-to-mouth motion habit is strong and doesn't go away easily. It is reminiscent of early childhood and the first way we learned. We picked up things and put them in our mouths. I had to retrain myself, first learning something different to do with my hands, then learning what to do with my hands that didn't involve eating. As an active person, I had to make a conscious effort NOT to play with my hair, pick at my skin and nails, drum my fingers, pull my ears, scratch or any of those horrible, annoying habits. It was difficult, but I finally adjusted to having my hands quietly in front of me or resting lightly on my hips.

The second part to quitting is letting go of the chemical addiction. I made it through this step with the help of nicotine gum. I chewed it whenever I had a craving for nicotine and then tapered off a little as I found substitutes for the social aspects. Quitting the gum and coping with my body screaming for nicotine was another story. I was in touch with my body's needs and it screamed for nicotine – for days. It takes dedication and willpower to get off nicotine. For me, it involved canceling everything and just going to bed until the screaming was over. Even now, I occasionally wake up in a cold sweat because I dreamt I started smoking again. Nicotine is the most addictive substance known to man. After fourteen years of NOT smoking, I still crave nicotine. This is the one exception to my rule of investigating cravings. Don't ever expect *that* craving to go away. And don't ever give in. One man I know said he started smoking again because he thought that one day he wouldn't want a cigarette. That day will *never* come.

I find I am a much more productive and happier person since I quit, and I still thank the people who encouraged and helped me.

So, treat your body like you love it. It will treat you the same way.

Chapter 5

The Magical Weight Loss
Elixir Is Sweat

I don't know who "they" are, but remember when they used to say, "Never let them see you sweat?" I don't know who "them" is, either. I am willing to bet that "they and them" are not interested in you personally; otherwise, "they" would not be giving you such bad advice. Maybe you don't want "them" to see you sweat, but you'd better see *yourself* sweat at least twice a week or you are asking for trouble. Besides, isn't calling someone "hot" a compliment?

Turn on the television or flip through a magazine and you'll see products that are advertised as "fat burners." The one true "fat burner" is oxygen. You can't buy it in a pill or drink it in a milkshake. It's been there for you the whole time. To get oxygen to burn fat you have to use up excess energy, and that means moving around, breathing and *sweating*.

Oxygen is one of the three components for burning everything, including fat. The process of burning is called *oxidation*. Heat, fuel and oxygen combined together make fire. It's pretty simple. A fire can't be sustained without all three ingredients – take any one away, and the fire goes out. Even rust is a form of oxidation, but technically, it's a slow burn.

If a person has excess energy to burn and breaks a sweat, but doesn't breathe properly, what have you got? Not fat-burning! If someone is breathing properly, has excess energy to burn, but doesn't break a sweat, there's no burning either. The last combination, when someone exercises and breathes with no fuel, is called anorexia. No thank you.

The main point I am trying to make is this: *Breathe as if your life depended on it*. By breathing correctly, breaking a sweat once in a while and giving your body the proper fuel, the only thing you've got to lose is excess weight.

Years ago, I took a scuba diving class. The instructor spent hours instructing us on proper breathing technique. Because we were underwater carrying our oxygen supply, we needed to learn how to conserve it, not waste it, through "shallow-breathing." While it may sound obvious, he wanted us to use every molecule of oxygen. By breathing slowly and deeply, every molecule of air would be absorbed and metabolized. He told us most people only breathe in the top third of their lungs. This means that two-thirds of an average person's lung capacity is wasted. To me, this means you can get three times the number of fat burners (oxygen molecules) working for you just by breathing right.

There is a lot of debate about fast metabolisms, slow metabolisms and whether they can change or not. My belief is that people *can* improve their metabolism by eating well and having a high activity level. I also believe that the reverse is true: People can damage their metabolism by eating poorly and being sedentary. I have read that researchers now believe a person can raise their metabolism by 1 to 2 percent and that even small increases in metabolism would make a major difference in the amount of energy used versus energy stored. When a small change in just the right area yields big results, it is called "leverage." Having leverage work for you, rather than against you, is the key to accomplishing great things. We'll talk more about it in Chapter 6 and Chapter14.

If you have been shallow breathing most of your life, this concept may seem a little strange. The first thing to do to "raise" your metabolism is to get that fire inside of you up to a roaring blaze. So sit up straight and *practice* moving air in and out of your body. Make sure you give your lungs some breathing room – breath in deeply from your nose, feel it moving down to your waist, hold for a second, then push the air back up and out of your body. Try it lying down. Place your hands on your stomach and feel it rise and fall as you slowly take in long, deep breaths and let them out again. You can feel your abdominal muscles pushing out that stale air to let in the good stuff that you *really* need. Trust me, it sounds basic, but it's the only way to get this process moving.

Many activity disciplines highlight this breathing process. It is especially important in yoga, where proper breathing and flexibility activities are used to decrease stress and increase spiritual harmony. I use a few yoga techniques in my own personal workout routine.

Remember the next part for building that fire? Fuel? It's all about proper nutrition and ensuring you receive the right vitamins and minerals. If there's not enough iron in the blood, a person feels exhausted. Iron (a mineral) holds oxygen in the blood cells and comes from dark green vegetables, eggs, soybeans, lean beef, fish and baked potatoes or mineral supplements. An iron molecule is an iron molecule. Your cells don't care which source they get it from. When you have enough iron in your blood cells to carry enough oxygen to your other cells, your metabolism kicks into high gear and you feel great. Your bloodstream (along with other systems) also carries every nutrient that your body needs to repair itself, think your thoughts and take you where you want to go. This is called "metabolization." Literally, it is the maintenance of life – your life. Scientifically, it is the building up and breaking down of living cellular material, along with *a corresponding expenditure of energy*.

Now, think about what you see when you look at a fire. Oftentimes, when you see smoke rising from a fire, you think of the air pollution it is creating. Just as a fire causes exhaust, smoke or pollutants to rise from a smokestack, your internal fire, or metabolism, causes cells to use fuel and discard pollution. The cells use oxygen to oxidize and the leftovers are oxidants. This is where more vitamins and minerals come in. The cell pollution binds with anti-oxidants and leaves your body as waste while your kidneys and liver clean your blood. Incredible, isn't it?

Once again, think back to that fire. Have you ever tried to light a fire by holding a match right up to the fireplace log? Did it work? Probably not. You must have some kind of kindling to get the burning started. If you had a load of lumber and no kindling, newspapers or lighter fluid, you'd stay pretty cold. For the body, that necessary kindling or starter is a carbohydrate.

I have no idea how carbohydrates (or starches) got the bad reputation they have today. They come in many different, marvelous forms: breads, potatoes, cereals, rice, sugars, fruits and vegetables. I can't live without them. Carbohydrates are instant energy, just like kindling. They provide your body with calories. Calories are simply a measure of a unit of heat. This is what your body burns when it breathes, thinks, talks and moves around. I eat carbohydrates about five times a day to make sure I've got high quality fuel.

The starches in carbohydrates are broken down and turned into simple sugars by the saliva in your mouth and are moved along by your digestion system. So, why not just swallow the contents of the sugar bowl? While plain white sugar is a carbohydrate, it only gives you empty calories: energy, but no nutrition. I dislike an empty calorie like I dislike an empty gift box in a store display. So very disappointing!

Sure, we sometimes want that piece of chocolate cake or a sweet soda. That's fine. Just don't make those empty calories your staple foods. Many people substitute fake sugars in the sugar bowl. I stay away from substitutes like NutraSweet ®, Equal ®and Splenda ® because they give me a headache. Besides, I don't know what is in them and I don't want to be shortchanged. I *hate it* when someone automatically gives me a diet soda because I am thin. I did not get thin by drinking diet soda and I don't know anyone who ever did and lived to tell the tale!

I don't know if you have noticed by now, but one of my big, skinny secrets is this: I try to take care of my spine and my circulation system. I choose my activities, exercises and foods with their benefits in mind. If those two parts of me are in good shape, everything else will follow, such as glossy hair, a toned stomach and smooth thighs. That means exercising, getting enough sleep and eating right nine days out of ten. This provides me with reserves, both mental and physical, so I can take on whatever comes my way. I have my life arranged so that eating well and exercising is easier, cheaper and more fun than sitting on my duff and calling the Pizza Palace day after day. (By the way, I think pizza is nature's perfect food.) And I am certain that you can do the same in your life. It will make you happier, healthier and centered.

Now that you've heard enough on nutrition, let's move on to exercise: What it is, what it isn't and how you can work it in to benefit *you.*

Have you ever heard the saying, "No Pain, No Gain?" It's a lie. I think the saying should be "No Sacrifice, No Gain." A sacrifice doesn't necessarily have to hurt. Although we make some sacrifices willingly, there is *always* a choice involved. You have to give up something when you make a sacrifice. There is *always* something else that we can be doing or eating or saying or thinking.

So, I sacrifice some TV and arguing time to exercise. I like to exercise until I smile. Exercising releases chemicals called endorphins that put me in a good mood that lasts all day. If you are exercising until you hurt, you are doing too much.

I don't worry about cardio versus weight training or whether my heart rate is at the right level. I just get my blood pumping and my body moving. It is through this, even as a mother in my late 40's, that I am still the same 119 pounds with perfect cholesterol and blood pressure levels as I was at twenty.

Benefits

You have already heard of the benefits of exercise, but I'm going to give you a few more to consider.

Exercise reduces the level of fat in the abdomen and can prevent the development of serious medical conditions such as diabetes and heart disease. Heart disease is the number one killer in the United States. Diabetes can cause blindness and can reduce circulation in the legs – extreme cases can lead to amputation. In some communities, *more than half* of all health problems are weight related.

Exercise helps the body eliminate toxins more efficiently. Fluid retention causes pain by restricting oxygen to the brain and the abdomen. Exercise helps balance fluctuating hormone levels for people who suffer from PMS. It actually is *proven* to lift depression for some people better than medication.

You have to do a combination of both "strength training" and "aerobic" (or "cardio") activities to get the full benefits of exercise. The aerobic/cardio exercises strengthen your circulatory system and strength training keeps your muscles and bones in top condition. Unfortunately, you have to do *both* to be in good shape or for weight loss to occur. It doesn't happen if you only do one.

Exercise causes muscle mass to increase and causes your metabolism to rise. Because resting muscle uses more energy than working fat, it uses more oxygen, which leads to more fat burning. A friend of mine who had never exercised and had always been shocked by my appetite began a cardio and strength-training program. After a few months and dropping more than a dress size, she said, "I finally understand how you could always eat so much!" It just proves a little change in her activities allowed her to change her metabolism and helped her to be happy in her own skin. If she can do it, you can, too. I think you *can* change your metabolism.

There is a paradox to this, however. Because muscle weighs more than fat, an in-shape person can weigh more than a similarly sized out-of-shape person. That's why I don't advocate a daily weigh-in. It would be easy to get discouraged if you made a lot of changes only to see the scale numbers creeping up. It's much better to gauge your weight by how you look and feel than by the numbers, especially if you are like many people and let one bad factor outweigh a host of good factors. If you must use a measurement, find an old pair of jeans. Put them on in the morning once a week and feel them loosen up as your muscles tone and your fat level falls.

Flexibility is another benefit to exercise. Joints don't have their own circulation system and must rely on the movement of muscles and bones to circulate blood and lymph into the sacs between them. These sacs (called bursa or discs) are filled with thick fluid to cushion the spaces where your bones meet. Without circulation, the bursa can wither and die, causing intense pain. The pain causes the nearby muscles to freeze up, further shutting down the circulation in a vicious cycle that can lead to permanent damage. This is why the treatment for those who have "thrown out" their backs is moderate movement to keep the circulation going, rather than bed rest, which would make the damage worse.

Have you heard the old wives tale that you should wait an hour after eating before swimming for fear of getting a cramp? People get cramps from a lack of potassium, not from moving after eating. Exercise actually *alleviates* cramps. Do any of us get cramps at all within one hour of eating? Are people walking down the street doubled over in pain? I don't see people leaving restaurants with cramps. What about biking or walking? I think right after eating is the perfect time to go for a walk or a bike ride. Maybe people who get cramps after eating still belong to the Clean-Plater Club.

So what is exercise anyway? It's *anything* that gets your circulation going and your muscles moving.

What's Your Routine?

You know the benefits. Now, what do *you* do for exercise? In years past, people got exercise in their daily lives. They didn't even have to think about it. They hoed gardens, lifted bales of hay, and rode horses. Sausage was invented to give these folks extra calories just to make it through the day. They walked *everywhere* they wanted to go. We don't.

I once had a roommate who made breakfasts of sausages, bacon, grits, and pancakes every morning. Then she would complain that people made fun of her about her weight. I pointed out that perhaps it might have something to do with what she ate every morning. She said to me "But, Ces, I'm a country cook!" I countered: "But, Debbie, you don't plow the lower forty or stack hay bales every day. You drive to work and sit at a desk when you get there." She did *not* get the connection. Later, she went on the "Poverty Diet." It works like this: If you don't have any money to buy food, you don't eat, so you lose weight. Although she had lost much of her extra weight, she had badly ridged fingernails and a pallor complexion that may have been caused by protein and vitamin deficiencies. She looked awful! I don't know if her weight loss lasted and I *really* don't recommend it as a weight loss strategy.

Before taking drastic measures, look at what you do every day and ask yourself, "What *is* my routine?"

There are a lot of little things that I do every day because they have become my routine; they give me energy and make me feel healthy. My routine is simple. I *never* take the closest parking space. I always leave it for those who really need it. I feel sorry for the folks who sit in their cars with the engines running until a close parking space becomes available. Is it painful for them to walk? Are they lazy? Or, are they just not thinking? The funny thing is, I usually make it into the building before they do! Every time I park my car I have another reason to be happy that I'm healthy. I get the satisfaction of feeling generous, *and* a little bit of exercise. And my trade-ins are worth more because I have less door dings from shopping carts and tightly parked cars. It is something simple anyone who drives can do every day.

Another easy way to sneak in exercise is climbing two flights of stairs. When faced with a choice of the elevator or stairs, I always go for the stairs if it is one or two flights – *no matter what I'm carrying*. If I carried it into the building, I'll carry it up the stairs. If I'm going to the fourth floor, I usually go for the elevator but I make an effort to walk back down. Would you believe that people pay big money to use stair-stepping machines? In most buildings they're right in front of you for free. I think there should be bulletin boards on the walls in stairwells. There are all kinds of neat posters in elevators, but I usually have to get out before I've read them; people can get so touchy when you hold the elevator.

You can get a good workout doing the things you do on a daily basis and you don't even have to do leg lifts while you brush your teeth. I learned this from a friend when I watched her pick up her two-year-old. She didn't bend over him; she kept her back straight and squatted down next to him, then lifted him up with her legs, like a weightlifter. I talked to her a little bit and, sure enough, she lifted weights a couple of times a week. I was so impressed; I quit my gym and joined hers because the child-care was better. Any time you have a chance to pick something off the ground, you can do a squat. For me that's about 25 a day.

I also have a little floor exercise routine that takes five minutes (or less) in the morning. I stretch, do some upper crunches, lower crunches, five "boys" push-ups and five reverse sit-ups. I don't even do it every day. All I need is 90 seconds and a space on the floor to be able to hit the shower saying "Not too shabby!"

Other parts of my routine include walking my dog around the block, riding my bike when I need to relax and playing great games of tag with my daughter and her friends. One of her friends said, "My mom never plays with us like this!" I think that is sad in two ways: Her mom is missing out on valuable time with her child *and* she's missing a great opportunity to exercise. How many calories do I burn? I don't have a clue, but I have fun doing it and the kids know I care about them.

I used to have heavy-duty hobbies like snow skiing and scuba diving. There is nothing to keep you in shape like heaving 100 pounds of equipment onto your back and throwing yourself into rough seas. Unfortunately, marriage and motherhood don't leave much time for pursuing these anymore, so I have to get my exercise by other means.

One unexpected area to work out in is in the garden. I garden like crazy. Trimming trees, moving mulch, and digging in the dirt are fantastic ways to stay in shape. It also gives you something to show for it when you're done. I even sponsored a gardening club at my daughter's elementary school, spending an hour a week and inspiring the kids to take on things they never dreamed they would. I changed their lives and they changed mine.

If you like to garden, there are plenty of community centers and schools that would love to have a garden sponsor.

Call up the local nursery or home improvement store. They'll donate plants in exchange for a small sign recognizing them for their generosity and you'll be on your way. Just be ready to get your hands dirty. Oh, and get some cheap magnifying glasses for the kids. Triple bonus! You get a work out, the community gets a garden and some kids get individual attention, as well as a science lesson. What more could you ask for?

If you don't like to garden, there are all kinds of established programs that don't have enough adult volunteers. City recreation centers, Girl and Boy Scouts, Little Leagues and schools can all use people to continue their good work. Just don't sit around and watch. You can easily trade one or two hours of your time a week for a workout and help your community, too.

Our kids need more attention than they are getting right now. Our society has given up the "stay-at-home parent" without substituting alternative "parenting." Many families have not replaced the important efforts that went into the home that now are going into the workplace instead. I think the issue of disadvantaged children is not about money anymore. The "haves" these days are the children who get attention. The "have-nots" are the ones who get ignored.

What has this got to do with exercise? You can step into the breach. You can get up off the couch and shoot hoops at the rec center. You can be an assistant coach for Little League or an assistant Scout Leader. You can help organize walk-a-thons: just make sure to walk. No one cares if you are any good – just show up dressed and ready to play the game. You can fill two voids at once. You can replace activities you are missing and give attention to someone who really needs and deserves it. You have nothing to lose (but weight) and everything to gain.

Often, people automatically get out and do many outdoors activities in the summer, but when winter arrives, it takes some thought to get moving. One way to solve this problem was mentioned before – get comfortable in a sporting goods store. Pick out something you would like to do and fit it into your routine. Don't wait until you have time to exercise – that is denial of the first degree. You will *never* have time unless you make it happen. Schedule your exercise routine into your busy week. By trying different things, you won't get bored and you'll become more interesting to be around – both to yourself and to others. Again, check with your doctor before you make changes to see if the changes are right for you.

My Only Gold Card is to the Gym

If I can't get outside to exercise, I use my only Gold Card and go to the gym. I will always belong to a gym, even if I don't go for months at a time. Some people may feel uncomfortable thinking about all the hard-bodies you see on TV commercials. But there is a gym for everybody. Some cater to women. Others accommodate bodybuilders, new mothers, older folks, single professionals… You get the picture. There is a gym for you – you just need to look for it.

Many gyms are full of a bewildering array of equipment that resembles a medieval torture chamber. There are free weights, lifting machines, Stairmasters, treadmills – all kinds of weird stuff. But, like anything else, it's only overwhelming until you understand what the equipment is and how to use it.

The equipment is basically divided between weight training and cardio. Weight training strengthens your muscular and skeletal systems and the cardio strengthens your cardiovascular system. Huh? Translation: The weights are for your bones and muscles and the treadmills are for everything else. You lift the weights with various parts of your body for a certain number of times ("or reps") that make up something called a "set" for "strength training" your muscles. Most people lift weights in sets of eight to twelve reps.

The treadmills and Stairmasters are for "cardio." In other words, by moving your muscles, you get the heart pumping large amounts of oxygen-rich blood to all of your organs, which strengthens your heart and helps it move the good stuff in and the bad stuff out of your three hundred trillion cells. Your brain gets a huge dose of oxygen and you can think more clearly, making your problems less insurmountable.

Current research indicates that you receive 90 percent of the benefits of exercise from the first "set" of strength training.

So why bother with the second? For me, I don't see much extra benefit. One set of twelve reps is usually all I do. If you want to do more sets, go ahead – just be careful not to overwork your muscles. Otherwise, do one set and get a workout completed in less than an hour.

My usual activities keep me in pretty good shape most of the time. When I am feeling out of shape, I will go to the gym twice a week for about three months for a tune up. This is my little exercise routine when I go to the gym:

First, I warm up on the stationary bike. Sometimes I read, but most often I just think. Then I stretch for a few minutes. Next, I do something called circuit training. I have been doing this off and on for more than thirty years and it works just as well now as it did when I began.

Basically, you go from one piece of equipment to the next and exercise each part of your body. As you move around the circuit, the part that was exercised rests while you exercise the next part. The machines are even numbered. Start at one and move to two, etc. You don't have to think about it and you *can't* do it every day because your muscles must rest for a day to rebuild. Twice a week is plenty. You can get great results in just a few weeks if you don't hurt yourself and give up.

It drives me crazy when I see people bouncing from one machine to another across the room and not "doing the circuit." They are not helping themselves at all.

Some people think they have to look good to go to the gym. There *are* people who will get ready to exercise as if they were going out for the evening. Teased hair, gold chains: and those are the men. You won't be putting your self-esteem on the line in front of them. They won't even notice you. They are so into *themselves* and how they look, you won't even appear on their radar screen. It *is* pretty neat, however, when you *are* looking good and they *do* notice you. At that point you can pretty much say to yourself, "I'm feeling good and looking good, I can go on to other things now." Or, you can *join* them.

My At-Home Routine

I think everybody needs an at-home routine they can do regularly. You may not make it to an exercise appointment, but if you can take two or three minutes before you start your day, you won't have to live with the guilt. Warm up for every day like you would any other physical activity. Athletes warm up before working out and competing and you have important work to do today, too. They have great bodies and so can you. Just a little stretching to warm up, a little strengthening for a couple of minutes, some cool down and you're set.

Start any way you want, but the idea is to get the circulation going between your bones, and then strengthen some key muscles, especially the ones that don't get any exercise during the rest of your day. For me, that's my back and my abdomen.

To start, find a clear spot on the floor with either carpeting or a mat. Bend down, let the top of your head hang towards the floor, put your hands behind whatever you can reach: ankles, knees or thighs and pull gently two or three times for two or three seconds. This loosens up your spine and allows the circulation to get into the joints between the vertebrae in your back. Clasp your hands together, straighten up and stretch your arms over your head. Then bring your arms slowly down to your side. This will loosen up your shoulders. Roll your head in a circle to release the tension in your neck. There are all kinds of great exercise books and magazines available to get ideas on how to tailor a warm-up to your own needs.

Many times when people exercise, they try to "spot reduce" a problem area, such as the thighs or buttocks. You can't "spot reduce" any more than you can use gas from one part of a full tank, but you can "spot tone" these areas. By exercising certain muscle groups you can tighten them and push fat out of the way. Consider the abdominals, for instance.

We have *both* upper abdominal and lower abdominal muscle groups. Therefore, we have to do *two* types of abdominal exercises to tighten up those muscles and push away that fat. These exercises are called "crunches."

Upper crunches are for the group just under the ribs. You lie on the floor with your knees up and feet flat on the floor and relaxed. Put your hands behind your neck, sort of like the sit-ups they used to make you do in gym class, and lift your chin toward the ceiling. Your head should lift off the floor about four or five inches. It's harder than it sounds and it's *enough*. I do between five and twelve, depending on how much time I've got.

I do a second type of upper crunch for my waist. While lying on the floor, put your left ankle lightly on your right knee. With your hands behind your neck, try to touch your right elbow to your left knee. This is also harder than it sounds. I do between five and twelve of these and then switch sides and do between five and twelve more.

Lower crunches are easier. Lie on the floor with your arms out in a "T" shape and just pull in your legs until your knees are touching your chest. Then straighten your legs again. I try to keep my feet just lightly grazing the floor, but if you have to walk your legs in and back out again – at least you have a start.

Unless you are in top shape, DO NOT try the leg lifts you did in high school without the help of a professional trainer. These are when you lift your legs until your toes are pointed to the ceiling and then lower them slowly. You will hurt and possibly permanently injure your back because all of your weight presses on two or three little bones in your spine. There is little wonder why there are so many back problems these days because we *all* did them.

Lastly, with my arms still outstretched, I pull my knees up to my chest and slowly rock from one side to the other a few times. It is like a back massage for one. With my legs up, the small of my back rests directly on the floor and I can feel every joint in my spine loosening up and getting the circulation it needs. Wonderful!!

Just like the abdomen, you can spot tone the backs of your arms through simple floor exercises. "Boys" push-ups are when you are face down on the floor, with your palms pressed against the floor at your shoulders and your weight on your toes. Keeping your back straight – don't sway your back or lift your butt up – straighten your arms to go up and then bend them to touch your nose to the ground. Repeat this a few times. "Girls" push-ups are when you have your knees on the ground instead of your toes. If you need to, start with these and eventually work your way up to the "boys" method. When done correctly, these strengthen *everything*.

The ideal is to be able to complete a whole set of push-ups. But let's get real. It doesn't matter how you start to heave yourself into the air, only that you start. If, on the first day, you can only manage to push up your head and part of your chest, it's a start. You'll do better later. Don't beat yourself up about it.

If I have time, I do a couple of "reverse sit-ups" on my Roman chair, but if not, I do five or six by hooking my legs under my dresser. I can finish in less time than it took you to read this.

I find that if I do this routine between two and four times a week, my other weekly activities will keep the rest of me in shape.

Cool Down

Cool down is a short period of slower moving activity performed before you get to fall on the couch and rest. If you have done what you need to do for exercise (in addition to your at-home routine), you have worked up at least a moderate sweat: the magical weight-loss elixir. You now need to cool down before sitting down. During exercise, your three hundred trillion cells have been oxidizing like mad and throwing off pollution. Some of this pollution is called lactic acid and will cause sore muscles if you don't move it out of your body after exercise. If you have ever had a "stitch" or pain in your side, you know what I mean.

Have you ever heard the expression, "Rode hard and put away wet" in regard to something haggard or worn out? It has to do with horses. If a horse is put into the stable after a ride without cooling down, it will become very sickly. You don't want to do that to yourself, either. If you watch sprinters, they don't stop and fall down at the finish line. They run right past it and then keep walking for a minute or two to let the lactic acid move out of their muscles. You *must* do the same before resting; otherwise you will feel awful later, blame it on the exercise and then give up.

What is Exercise, Anyway?

I like to look at exercise as "activity." Getting up and moving around needs to be enjoyable, otherwise we won't do it. We need to have activities that we can do for the rest of our lives that are going to fill our need for exercise. Think back to the things that you enjoyed in childhood. There are dozens of fun activities that qualify as exercise, but are not as boring as walking on a treadmill.

You do, however, need to draw a distinction between activities that condition you and activities that wear you out. So many people think that they get exercise from housework. It just wears me out. I don't know anybody who stays in shape just by doing housework. There are books that will tell you the "proper" way to get a housework workout. No thanks. I'd rather just get it over with and do something else. That's way too boring for me.

Dancing is exercise. Every professional dancer is in top shape. You don't have to be in top shape, just move around to the beat of the music. Think you can't do it? Even cowboys toss some corn meal on a slab of cement, put on a boom box and do the Texas Two-Step in their cowboy boots. There must be a hundreds of different dance classes you can sign up for – even if you're by yourself. I've set up my own, private disco in my garage with a mirrored ball and everything. It's pleasurable, it's satisfying and it's exercise!

Going somewhere is exercise. If travel agents put a package together and sell tickets for an activity, it's probably some kind of exercise. Think about it. Golf, tennis, walking tours – they are all forms of exercise.

Boating is great exercise. Sailors rarely need to exercise because the swaying of the boat causes their muscles to tense and relax constantly to stay at equilibrium. They are exercising and don't even know it.

We all hear about people who go for two-mile runs or do one hundred stomach crunches before breakfast. It seems like they had to get up at four o'clock in the morning to fit it in. Did you ever stop to think exactly how long it really takes to run a mile or do a crunch?

Well, my car idles at seven miles an hour. If I take my foot off the brake, the car will go seven miles an hour without touching the gas. Believe me, even on a bad day, I can walk faster than my car can idle. That means I can go a mile in less than fifteen minutes without even running – so anyone can do a two-mile walk or run *in less than thirty minutes*. If you bike at fifteen miles an hour, a five-mile bike ride *takes twenty minutes*.

A stomach crunch takes just a little over a second to do. At that rate, you can do a hundred in two minutes – in less time than it takes to watch the commercials between TV shows. Wow, if you had six minutes, you could do three hundred! Then wouldn't *you* be the one impressing people?

My point is this: YOU DO HAVE TIME TO EXERCISE! What you don't have time for is illness at this stage of your life or later. The body you have won't last forever, so get moving, get out there and enjoy it now!!

Look around you. Would anyone be interested in taking a tour of your city or neighborhood? There has to be something that people would pay to do. Do you live near a lake, a river, a beach or the woods? On a ranch or farm? Close to the big city? My guess is that if you thought about it, you could think of a half-dozen fun and satisfying things to do in a two-mile radius. Go canoeing or kayaking. Hike through the woods. Walk along the beach or simply wander around your neighborhood and enjoy the different styles of houses or different trees in the yards.

If you have access to a yard, kids or other people, music, car or boat, or floor, you can exercise. I even keep a list of parks in my glove compartment and an old tablecloth in the trunk. When I pick up some fast food, I head to the nearest park to enjoy it, either by myself or with a load of kids, instead of gulping it down in the car. They get to blow off some energy, and

I get to relax *or* join them. And I have *no* guilt about picking up fast food.

Go to the local park and act like a kid again. If I wasn't in shape or if I were recovering from an injury, the first thing I would do is hop on a swing and start swinging. You have to sit up straight. Try slouching and swinging – you won't be able to do it. Get your legs pumping, then your arms, and have fun. All the big muscles will start working and you can breathe from the bottom of your lungs. When you get going, you'll be able to feel the air in your hair and filling your lungs. It takes about two seconds to swing back and forth. You can do it a hundred times in less than five minutes. Go ahead and try it. It's low-impact, it's exercise and it's great fun.

If I were *really* out of shape, I would also get one of those tension bars that can be installed in a doorway. I would pull on it a few times a day to work my arm and rib muscles. Those are the ones you need if you ever lose your balance.

If none of those ideas work for you, here is a list of activities to get you started. Hopefully you'll add some more of your own.

These ARE Exercise

Yoga
Stretching
(Safely) Lifting and carrying boxes, coolers, groceries, children
Trimming trees, carrying the branches
Hide and Go Seek
Digging a flower garden
Riding a bike
Tennis
Swinging on a swing
Mowing the lawn by walking
Working out with weights
Playing outside until somebody squeals or laughs out loud
Walking
Hop Scotch

Jogging/Running
Kick the Can
Basketball
Singing
Playing on the monkey bars
Dancing: any kind
Carrying boxes to the attic
Jump rope
Swimming
Scuba Diving (one of my family favorites)
Walking the dog
Boating
Hula Hoop
Base-running
Kickball
Camping
Washing an active dog
Ice Skating
Volleyball

I used to like to:

1. _____

2. _____

3. _____

I have a place on the floor to stretch out: Yes_____ No _____

I have a towel or mat to stretch out on: Yes_____ No _____

I might like to try: _____

The nearest park is: _____

I have an old tablecloth in the trunk: Yes_____ No _____

These are NOT Exercise or Simply Wear You Out

Dusting
Paying bills
Vacuuming
Laundry
Card games
Cooking
Watching TV
Reading
Sitting
Writing
Driving
Talking on the phone
Grocery shopping
Riding a lawn mower
Computer work and games
Homework
Video games

I think the sum of all this is for you to "burn fat," you just need to eat a high quality meal (kindling), get up and do something that will get your heart pumping, (heating up and adding oxygen) and then keep doing it until some fat stores (logs) are tapped. Then stop, cool down and enjoy the good feelings. What else could there be?

One more thing to think about: Have you ever known someone who was confined to a wheelchair and couldn't walk? Wouldn't it be a miracle if they could get up and run? I think the answer is yes. Why is it any less of a miracle that *you* can do it? Appreciate what you have. Life's a game. Get in it.

Chapter 6

Healthy Is Sexy

There are many forms of health and they are all sexy. By sexy, I mean *really* attractive to other people – not superficial appearances that are deceiving. Physically healthy people have a lot of energy and are fun to be around. Mentally healthy people are the kind who "have it all together." Emotionally healthy people are well grounded and can be in give and take relationships – you both get something out of interacting with each other. Spiritually healthy people have found their place in the world and make you feel good just to be in their presence. I don't think a person can live a rich and fulfilling life if they are aren't healthy in all four areas.

At the risk of oversimplifying, I am going to separate the types of health and their manifestations into four categories. Physical health, of course, has to do with outward appearances. Because mental health manifests itself in behavior, that section will deal with functioning in everyday life. The section on emotional health will discuss feelings and their appropriate expression. The spiritual health section will deal with peoples' attitudes about themselves, the world and how they connect.

Over the years, as a beauty, clothing and financial professional, I have been in a position of trust for hundreds of people. You can really learn a lot about a person when you take off all their make-up in public, aid them in the fitting room, or delve into their personal finances. I found that many people do not draw a distinction between what they look like (physical), how they perform (mental), how they feel (emotional), and who they are (spiritual). Understanding how you perceive *and* present yourself are two major keys in getting what you want out of life.

These four types of health are so interconnected and interwoven into your life that you may not see them as distinct aspects of yourself. I liken them to four wheels on a car. You can't get the best performance if even one of them is a little low, but you can't pump air into one and expect it to get to the others. The good news is that because of this interconnectedness, a little maintenance in one area will have positive effects in all of the others. Although you might think a little effort will help only one area, you can leverage your efforts into all kinds of better health.

Notes on "The System"

I love to understand systems and how they work. My dad was a "systems analyst" for the military and I still remember him laughing when I said I was a "systems analyst" of life.

We all live in a complex web of systems. Our bodies are made up of atoms that mimic the form of the solar system. Our cells are little bodies of water with the same concentration of chemicals as the ocean. We live in social systems and have belief systems to explain how the world works. We are products of the education system. We use the monetary system. We work in an economic system. And we pay into the tax system for our governmental systems. Not only do we *exist* in systems, our *existence* is a system. So what do these systems have to do with physical, mental, emotional and spiritual health? E*verything*!!

If you don't understand and work with the systems in *your* life, sooner or later you are heading for a mental or physical catastrophe. The key to every kind of health is realizing what you are doing and what it is doing *for* you. You need to know how to work the system and how to make it work for you.

We all know people who faced enormous obstacles in life. We've seen them cope with those situations, move on and triumph when others would melt into a puddle. They have this remarkable inner strength, courage and power that comes from knowledge. They have belief systems that sustain them when everything appears to be working against them. They can look death in the eye and not flinch. It's not because they are fearless, it's because they know that they can *deal*!

Death can be the physical loss of someone or the loss of a relationship. In the first chapter, I talked about denial as the first step in the grieving process. People grieve for many reasons. They lose family members and friends. They lose loves. They lose jobs, and often their identity. I gave up my high level job and my fancy office to take on the hardest job I've ever had: motherhood. For a time, I grieved for the perceived loss of status in my life, but I accepted the change and tried to be the best mom I could be. I was still the same person in the power suit at the office as I was in slacks in the carpool, but I hated it when people treated me differently.

Healthy people quickly get over denial and deal with their grief, and the anger that comes with it, but in *constructive* ways.

By understanding the system, they know which resources they have to call on to make the best of the situations. Knowing how "the system" works will not make your life a bed of thornless roses. It will, however, let you know where to find the pliers to pull out the thorns that come your way.

A lot of people overeat or use other self-destructive habits to fill legitimate voids in their lives. The following sections can help you find inspiration to make positive changes in the daily habits that make up your life. Some of these sections will have *nothing* to do with food, but will have *everything* to do with changing how you feel about yourself.

Physical Health and Attractiveness

Every so often, fashion designers and make-up artists come up with a look that falls flat on its face. *Nobody* adopts it or buys the products associated with it. The latest was a hollow-eyed look the magazines called "heroine-chic." There may be a few who are attracted those who appear as if they will self-destruct, but most of us are *really* attracted to those who exhibit exuberant health. Most people are also "turned off" by signs of poor health. And history shows us the reason for this...

"Evolutionary psychologists" and "sociobiologists" study the *current* actions of people and relate them to past human species survival. They have found that the perceived attractiveness features of both males and females are indicators of good reproductive health. In other words, on a primal level, people are attracted to indicators of health because, by finding a healthy mate, a person's genetic material is more likely to be passed on in future generations. Those of us without children have time to pass on other great works to the future. But for most of us, having children is as close to immortality as we will get.

We are drawn to the healthy among us. It's no coincidence that most people first focus on another's eyes. Not only are they windows to the soul: they instantly reveal whether an individual is healthy. Teeth are a second indicator of good health. It's no coincidence that a beautiful smile is on everyone's top 10 list of attractors. We can't help it. Recent research has shown that tooth and gum problems can allow many kinds of germs to enter the blood stream and actually *cause* a number of illnesses that had never before been associated with the health of the mouth. A bright smile is pretty because it's *healthy*.

Skin is another organ associated with good health. Smooth, glowing, *touchable* skin is highly attractive to everybody. A flat stomach is another major indicator of good health. A distended belly is a symptom of many illnesses, both current and future. Fluid or fat accumulating in the gut can shorten a person's lifespan.

Whether we like it or not, others can garner reliable information about us based on our appearance. If they have nothing else to go on, potential mates can't help but pass on by if they notice signs of poor health. There are two reasons.

First, it is much easier to share child rearing with a healthy, long-lived mate rather than face the challenges of single parenting. Second, a healthy mate will be more likely to produce healthy offspring who will live longer to reproduce even more genetic material.

Another consideration for men is that a woman with a thick waist might already be in a committed relationship with another man. Wedding bands and pregnancy tests are a new invention as far as human history goes. I really think most men don't care whether their women are big or small, short or tall: they are just looking for someone with a waist smaller than her hips. No one should blame them for that.

The good news is that if we want to be physically attractive, eating well and getting active are the fastest ways to accomplish that goal.

Looks Aren't Everything

It's important to feel attractive. No one should feel badly because they want to dress up once in a while. People who think we should all look "natural" drive me crazy. But on the other hand, people are so much more than their looks.

Don't make the mistake of letting how you look be a measure of your worth to yourself and others. People get clues to others' personalities and abilities by their appearance. No one has time to get to know everybody they interact with on a daily basis. This is the reason I advocate that last look in the mirror before you head out the door. Often, the quality of our days depends on how we present ourselves. Life is a lot easier if our looks and personality match up.

But, it is a terrible mistake to think that what you *look like* is what you *are like*. Outsiders will look at you and judge you by the way you look. Do not make the same mistake. How you look indicates how you *feel*, not who you *are*. Don't confuse what you look like with who you are.

If you look good, it can give you confidence, and that is very attractive, but it doesn't make you a good person. Conversely, looking bad doesn't make you a bad person, but it does color the way you feel about yourself. Losing interest in one's appearance is a sign of depression and other mental ills. Also, eating something or other doesn't make you a bad person either, unless of course, you stole it.

For decades, every advertisement had a blonde-haired and blue-eyed model. Many people were convinced that if they didn't look like that, they weren't attractive. Our public standards of beauty have *finally* widened to accept many, many more people. I am so glad that dark-haired, red-haired, brown-eyed, Black, Asian, and Latin women have found their place in the Pantheon of Beauty. I have news for you women who never thought you were pretty: Your place is there, too. Get up there and take it.

Posture

I must have gotten my good posture obsession by seeing all those good-looking soldiers at bases around the world. And those on duty in Washington D.C. are the cream of the crop. I happened to be tutoring at my daughter's school in Florida, when there was a very important, unannounced visitor. I noticed a few extremely handsome men wearing earpieces and gleaming shoes. Looking around, I asked the principal why the Secret Service was at the school. He looked at me with shock and said that *no one* was to know of this visit until it was over, and asked me how I found out. I honestly didn't know anything about the visit, but it's a trademark of the Secret Service: Their clothes are perfect and they stand up tall.

Your mom had that right all along when she told you to stand or sit up straight. Think about what happens to your inner organs while you slouch in a chair. They are strangling. Bad posture can make you look *and* feel bad, and it coveys depression to others. It can also cause back, neck, shoulder, and head pain, and makes your digestion, respiratory and cardiovascular systems function inefficiently. That covers just about everything, doesn't it?

Even the Duchess of Windsor has one strategy we can borrow – her great posture. She may have only been trying to look regal, but a healthy body starts with good posture. It straightens your spine, gives your organs room to work and makes you look confident. People with good posture show the world that they matter. So sit up straight and breathe well. Practice a few simple back-strengthening exercises. All aspects of your health will benefit.

Mental Health and Attractiveness

Good mental health is the ability to function well in all areas of your life. It manifests itself in your behavior: how you perform. People who show up on time, spend money reasonably and take simple precautions in everyday life exhibit good mental health. These are the people with whom most of us want to have relationships.

People who need rescuing over and over can really drag you down. But, many of us do the same thing over and over because we are on autopilot. We *have* to be on autopilot in many respects because making decisions on mundane things day after day will leave you with no life to live. This is why have food jags and other responses that are automatic. For example, have you ever driven yourself home from work, but upon arrival, had no recollection of the journey? You were on autopilot. You had made that journey enough times until your unconscious could say, "I know where we are headed, I'll take over now." It doesn't only work with driving. You go on autopilot in many ways without even realizing it.

In Chapter 4, I talked about having items and activities that made weight control automatic for me. I don't need willpower: I just head for my bike instead of the fridge when I'm upset. They are only about twenty feet apart, but even that tiny distance, over years of time, has benefited me tremendously.

Choices

The choices you make every day need to be consciously made by you or you'll end up sleepwalking through life. Your choices allow you to live life on your terms. Your terms are your choices – if you don't make them yourself, they can't be yours.

Having no choices can be bad, but having unlimited choices can be bad too. With unlimited choices, it is possible to "overthink" and live in fear of making a mistake. Allow yours elf to make some mistakes – you'll learn from them. Just for a minute, turn off your autopilot. And do some arbitrary choosing of your own.

Saying "No"

Some people give an automatic "yes" response in every situation. You must be able to say "no" to keep yourself from getting overwhelmed. Learn to say "no" gracefully in about 10 different ways. Practice on the speaker box at the drive-through if you have to. You don't have to be mean, just firm enough for people to get the message. You may know people who do not take the first "no," or the second, so you need 10 on hand for all situations. Examples could be: "You've caught me at a bad time" and "I'm afraid I can't work it into my schedule." Any good etiquette book will have great suggestions on letting people down easy. You need to keep some "you" for you. If you let people down quickly and easily, they can then move on to get what they need from another relationship. You especially need to avoid an automatic "yes" when it comes to money.

Money

So many people make the wrong decisions day after day with their money. Magazines would have you believe that happiness is found in a store. But as every reformed Grinch knows, true happiness comes from within. Making money and spending money are two important functions in our society. Money, or the lack thereof, can affect you physically, mentally, emotionally and spiritually. By looking at money objectively, life won't be happier, but life will be easier and money will have less power over you.

With a financial plan, you will see the distinction between "making and spending" and the "use" of money. "Make and spend" connotes a lack of control: of course you want to spend your money. "Using" money implies having control over it. You might think twice about *spending* on an item if you don't want to *use* your money that way. And control is what it's all about, isn't it? Having things the way we want them?

You have a relationship with money and money "mediates" your relationships with other people: spouse, kids, parents, bosses and other co-workers, friends and strangers. Although you may not think about it, your interactions with others are affected by your use of money. Your relationships can be distorted through the money "prism." You may see yourself either richer or poorer than you really are and eventually, this distortion can cause a huge amount of stress in your life.

Having a good relationship with money is important for mental health. When money is short, everything seems like a crisis, but only a bump in the road when funds are plentiful. Ask anyone who has ever lost a job, or had a sick kid and no insurance, or a car to be repaired and bad credit.

Unfortunately, the three basic things you need for monetary peace of mind are *invisible*. You can't set them on a table like a sculpture and admire them, and it sounds crass when you talk about them. But like the roof over your head, you only notice the importance of financial security when the ceiling begins to leak on a rainy day. The three components of monetary peace of mind include insurance, good credit and savings.

Insurance

You can't look in the mirror and say to yourself, "Wow, my new insurance is really looking good today!" Insurance is a stated loss: you pay someone to assume your risk. You agree to lose a certain amount of money and the company will cover you in case of a health, home or automobile disaster. To minimize the cost, you must agree to take actions to minimize the chances of disasters, such as wearing your seat belt and not smoking. Having good insurance can make the difference between a peaceful life and a worrisome existence.

Credit

Good credit is essential *and* invisible. The trouble with a credit report is that it may be yours but you don't own it. You are not even allowed to see your report unless you get a "consumer copy" from a bureau. If you have a record of paying your bills on time and are not over-extended, you have a high credit score and are a low risk. If you are a slow-payer or a non-payer, you have a lower credit score and are a higher risk. If your automatic response is to whip out your credit card at every opportunity, you are probably in the second group. If you have good credit, you will pay less for items over your lifetime. You will then have more money to put in savings and invest, and more readily achieve the financial peace of mind that is essential to a balanced life.

Savings

Savings are also essential, but when you put money away, all you have is a number on a piece of paper: you don't have that cool new TV. Where is the satisfaction in that? It's no wonder people aren't saving their money. Head for the library and check out a personal finance book. You'll find many, many ways to establish a savings account, even if all you do is roll your change and deposit it every month. After you have a couple of thousand dollars saved up, you can look at other investments that have higher returns. If you are going to have a balanced life, I can't think of anything else that would be more satisfying than watching the numbers creep up on a bank statement. Most people are living from paycheck to paycheck and most people are overweight from stress eating – remember the rich and the thin? There's no coincidence there.

The Plan B Fund

Anybody who receives a W-2 at their job should have a *minimum* of three months expenses in cash – just in case. This money can be used if you get sick and can't work, if you get fired or laid off, or if you just get so frustrated you say, "I quit." People who work seasonally or are in highly paid executive positions should prepare for the possibility of being out of work for six months to two years. It may sound like a lot of money, but if your current job, Plan A, doesn't work out, having a Plan B fund will make it a lot less stressful. Once you have that money put away, then go out and get a new television or have a fancy meal. But make sure you create a fund – it will be a gift that money can't buy – peace of mind. You'll be more confident just knowing that it's there and that's *attractive*.

Emotional Health and Attractiveness

Is happiness a place? No, it's a state of being. But, how can you wrap your mind around a "state of being" if you aren't some sort of saint or guru? I decided for myself that happiness is the vehicle, not the destination. There are happy people and unhappy people in all walks of life. If people can be happy in all kinds of outside circumstances, then happiness *must* come from within. It must be a person's attitude toward circumstances: their feelings. When you have good emotional health, you experience your feelings instead of denying them. You express them in a way that attracts others. You can deal with them without being overwhelmed, and that takes self-esteem.

Self-Esteem

People with the best kind of emotional health have what I have come to call "deserved self-esteem." They have what it takes to take on life: the right attitude. They achieve their goals through hard work and perseverance. They can look at their lives for exactly what they are and find beauty in them.

There are also people with low self-esteem who should be proud of themselves. They just aren't for some reason. They can't seem to get a handle on things and aren't living to their full potential. Some people have low self-esteem for a reason. They really messed up somehow, but don't know how to go about fixing the situation. The good news is that if people want to change, they can. Sometimes it takes a lot of effort, but it can be worth it.

There are also people with "undeserved self-esteem." They have done very little with their lives but take advantage of unearned wealth, talent, or other people. I can write this without fear of retribution because not one of them will be reading *this* book. But don't be envious of them. There are so many instances of people who crash when they lose their looks or their family money. They haven't bothered to develop a personality to help them through the wrinkles and the rough spots when they come along.

Relationships

Whatever your goals are in life, they have to include other people – no one does it alone. Good health depends on cultivating good relationships. There are five fingers on each of two hands. Your choices are limited if you only have use of one finger.

But, first and foremost, you *must* have a good relationship with yourself before you can have solid relationships with others. You can't be all things to yourself, but you need to strive to be most things to yourself. When you know you can depend on yourself for many of your needs, you are one of the people with deserved self-esteem.

Managing Relationships

Many times we fall into relationships because they are easy. They are already there and we go into them without thinking about it. We don't think about what we need and whether or not we have what it takes for the other person: like getting a big dog if you have a teeny apartment. Sometimes it's worth it to move and sometimes it's not.

Decide on which relationships you want to nurture and manage them properly. There are calls to make, appointments to keep and letters to write. There are "I love you's" to exchange: little pieces of your marvelous self that need to be sprinkled around like magic fairy dust, nourishing the ones who need it like they need air to breath. You can't do that if your head is in the fridge.

The Players

There are thousands of books on relationships because relationships are the most fascinating subject known to humans. However, there are a few things a lot of them don't point out. For example, relationships are two-fold. There are the *people* in the relationship and there is the *relationship* itself. People bring parts of themselves to every relationship. Sometimes they are generous and sometimes they are stingy. If a relationship is having problems, the people in it can only change *what they bring to the relationship*. You can't change *the other person*.

If you are not getting what you need from a relationship, it is *your* job to address it. Point out what you need and make suggestions to rectify the situation. The other person can either take your suggestions or not. If the other party refuses to work with your suggestions and compromise, then *you* have to make the change. You need to change the relationship.

This concept occurred to me when, during the first part of our romance, I asked my husband if he would still love me if I did this or that. He answered, "I would still love you, but I would miss you."

When people struggle to make a relationship work, many use the term "unconditional love." I love many people unconditionally, but if you want to have a *relationship* with me, then I have conditions. Others call them boundaries or limits, but I don't like those terms because they are static, and relationships are never static. If you lie to me, cheat on me or try to manipulate me, I might miss you, but probably not. There are too many nice people available to spend time with. Many people believe they can treat family members poorly because of the concept of unconditional love. And they often get away with it for that reason. These people are users. You may still love them, but you don't need to spend time with them. If you recognize these people in your relationships, you need to make a change.

Communication Breakdown

Human feelings don't conform to laws of physics. People react to the same situation in very different ways. There is no equal and opposite reaction to every action. Over and over, I have seen two people look at the same situation and come away with completely opposite conclusions. It *has* to be due to differences in perception. After years of observation, I noticed that people who have been exposed to emotional traumas react in one of two ways. Either they shut down and ignore both their own feelings and those of the people around them, or they develop highly sensitive antennae. Those with the sensitive antennae can read a whole book into a single sigh or a glance. Those who tend to shut down need to be hit over the head to understand another's point of view.

Because just about everyone has suffered an emotional trauma at one point, it's important to know which kind of person *you* are. You also need to pay attention to the reactions of those who are closest to you. If you have antennae, remember that not everyone receives the same signals. You are on the Internet while others are reading smoke signals. Be gentle with them. Those of us who shut down need to understand that at some point, we need to open up and make a serious effort to understand others' feelings if we want to have decent relationships again.

I've also noticed that people seem to react in one of two ways if shown vulnerability by another. Some open their hearts and vow to do anything possible to help another in need. Even perfect strangers. Others lunge straight for the jugular if they sense vulnerability. One type is not necessarily better than the other. However, people with open hearts need to choose the objects of their affection wisely and, unless they want to meet everybody's needs but their own, realize that not everyone is worthy of sacrifice. Lungers should understand that sometimes it is in their best interest to fill a need, rather than exploit it, if they want to have lifelong relationships. I sometimes look at peoples' reactions early on so I can tailor my relationships and save myself a lot of heartache.

I believe my family should be treated with the most care and respect. And I expect the same from them. We don't save our manners for strangers. We are so polite at my house; we even say "please" and "thank -you" to the dog. If you give respect, but get none in return, make a change. If you give love, but don't feel loved back – GET OUT! Many people don't appreciate what they have in a relationship until they lose it. And it's important for people to gain appreciation sooner rather than later.

New Players

If you are not happy in your relationships, you need to widen your radar screen. I believe everything exists in the world that I need for a happy life. It's up to me to go out and get it. Something that might be impossible for me to achieve might be a snap for someone else. I just have to widen my radar screen to find those people. Millions of people deserve your time and attention, and you deserve theirs. But it only takes a few who are really close to you to have a good and satisfying life.

You know those e-mail chains that tell you how much luck you will have if you forward the message to this or that number of people? It's not *forwarding* the sappy e-mail to your friends. It's *the friends* that bring you luck.

In the art of Feng Shui, it is said that having all the stove burners going at the same time will bring luck. I'm sure at some point someone noticed a lucky person had all their stove burners going. But why was that? It's not about the burners. It's the fact that if you have all the burners of your stove on at once, then you probably have a lot of people to *cook* for, and *they* are the ones who will bring you luck.

But it's really not luck. It's having good and satisfying relationships with people you trust that make your life worth living. There may have been a time when you were used and abused by people, but it is up to you to set the conditions of your relationships. Will you have healthy give and take relationships, or will you endure use and abuse?

Consider this: Many women tend to go for flashy guys who first appear on their radar screens. They go after the guy with the red convertible, rather than thinking about buying one for themselves. Ladies, the men you're going to have a solid give and take relationship with will not be flaunting their wealth at the neighborhood bar – you have to dig these nice guys out. They don't *have* to be flashy to feel good about themselves or put on some other "manly man" show. But if your radar screen is only tuned to see the big flashes, that's all you're going to see.

Just as some women are attracted to flashes of money and power, some men have the same problem with women. They pant after high-maintenance glamour girls who may be beautiful, but *they are as hollow as their cheekbones*. They have little to offer except their looks. If a man can't look at a woman, who at some point, has dirt under her fingernails and a milk stain on her blouse and still think she is extraordinary, he is losing out.

The simplest way out of this is to *go* out. Find some interesting things to do. Someone will want to join you and it only takes one.

Asking for Help

Asking for help is a difficult thing for a lot of people. Many seem to think there is something wrong with them if they can't do it all. Or they think that another is weak for asking. These people won't give, and they don't take. Someone needs to teach them. If the give and take of your relationships is out of balance, here is a suggestion.

At goal setting seminars, people learn about S.M.A.R.T. goals. Your goal should be Specific, Measurable, Attainable, Reasonable and Time bound. When you ask for help, your request should have the same conditions. My experience is that people are willing and even eager to help me if I can explain exactly what I need from them and what their contribution could be. It's always time, money or energy. They can say yes or no to a reasoned request.

This method works for me in any relationship, whether it's day-to-day relationships with my family or co-workers or writing to Congress people to get safe, outdoor activities. You won't get good results if your requests are too urgent or panicky. No one wants to help a drowning person for fear of being pulled under, too. By the same token, when I give help – my time, money or energy – I set parameters for my contribution. No one gets me as an open-ended resource. I don't let others drain me dry.

When you start out on your goal, put it on paper. You should be able to recognize the parts you need to accomplish yourself and the parts you can delegate. It is so much easier to get good help and a good result if you take the time to apply the S.M.A.R.T. criteria to your request. If your needs are still not being met, you know what to do.

Counseling

Sometimes it takes a trained professional to help people gain a good perspective on their lives. Counseling is like hiring another parent to pinch-hit. We know we can't be all things to all people. We can't even be all things to one person. How are parents supposed to meet every emotional need of their child? Speaking with a trained counselor can help people fill those gaps by showing how to make concrete changes that will last the rest of their lives.

Spiritual Health and Attractiveness

Spiritual, mental and emotional health are closely aligned. While mental and emotional health can often be medically improved, there is no substitute for a belief system. Spiritual health gives people the confidence and peace of mind that stems from knowing you belong in the universe. It's what gives people a sense of belonging and a connection with every other human being. And everyone knows that confidence is sexy.

No one knows when he or she will leave this world. The spiritually healthy person can accept that death is only a move to another world. Because they have made the most of this life, they have nothing to fear from what comes next. Many people use religion as their gateway to spiritual health, and use their faith in God to find inner peace. Whether you are religious or not, you need to feel a sense of belonging to the human race, and to feel connected with the power of consciousness.

People crave human connections, and popular culture revolves around these connections. It's all about sharing experiences. Movies are shared experiences that make people feel a sense of belonging. The trouble is when people use TV and movies as a substitute for real human connections. You can't blame people for seeking these outlets because human connections ultimately cause pain of one sort or another. Either the person hurts you during the relationship, or you hurt in some way when the relationship is over. It's so easy to let someone else do the loving and the hurting. The problem is that you become just a by-stander when you give up the love and relationships to avoid the hurt. Never settle for anything less than true human connections. It's those relationships that make life worth living. Even though relationships end, the hurt eventually goes away, but the love remains forever.

There will be times when you will grieve over the loss of a relationship by either someone's physical death, the death of your close feelings, or when you are separated from situations or people you love. But the love does not change; it's the relationship that changes.

Don't turn to food in your time of grief. Accept your grief as part of who you are and as evidence of the great love of which you are capable. Take time to grieve and to think of ways you can honor your lost relationship. Self-destructive actions will only add fuel to your grief.

You can use your grief to make yourself stronger. A friend's father was dying of cancer. Each day she would jog to the hospital to see him, relying on exercise as an outlet for her emotions. Although there was nothing she could do to save him, she grew stronger and more confident, and he could go in peace, knowing that she could take care of herself.

Lastly, don't just love people for their performance. Love them for who they are as well. At work, they love you for what you do – not who you are. Mentally, it's refreshing to turn in a great performance. But it does nothing for you spiritually if you think that's all you or your loved ones are. This also means that you should love your body for itself – just as it is – not because it meets some arbitrary standard.

Generosity

Good and generous people get taken advantage of every day. There, I said it. It's true. Now what is your reaction to that? You have three options. First, never do anything good or generous. Second, be good and generous and let everyone take advantage of you. Or third, make a deliberate choice and a conscious decision to be a good and generous person, but recognize when you are being taken advantage of, and set limits or conditions on your relationship. Most spiritually health people choose the last option.

Or you can also decide that that it doesn't matter. For example, I was working with a group of terrific people who were rebuilding a homeless shelter. When I would discuss what we were doing with friends and co-workers, the overwhelming majority offered whatever help they could and the project was a great success. However, there were a few people that suggested our project would probably be trashed the next day; people who didn't deserve it would live there and on and on. And, you know, that may be true. But I had to decide that the chance that someone would take advantage of our generosity was not going to stop me from being the good and generous person that I strive to be.

And here I get a little selfish because *it did not matter* to me what the reaction was of the future residents. I did not do it for their appreciation. I hope living there will be a turning point in their lives and they will appreciate it, but no one has a guarantee of anything. I have already gotten enough out of it: the camaraderie of a whole lot of first class people and the satisfaction that I did what I could. It's going to keep me going for years.

Beauty Sleep

You might think that skimping on sleep won't hurt you, but you are missing out on a lot if you do. Here's why: It is not called "beauty-sleep" for nothing. Getting enough sleep is crucial for physical, mental, emotional and spiritual health. People may brag about getting by on four hours of sleep, but it will take its toll eventually. You are short-changing yourself and those around you by failing to get enough because the body restores, repairs and maintains itself in every way through sleep.

Physically, muscles and bones are built and repaired, and the immune system can recover from the day's onslaught. Children grow only when they sleep. It's not necessary to get a facelift to look more rested – just rest. Also, there have been studies linking sleep deprivation to obesity. According to the American Council on Exercise and the National Sleep Foundation, too little sleep can cause an over-production of otherwise helpful hormones, wreaking havoc on a metabolism. I haven't studied the research myself, but I can tell you that I have *never* hit the snooze button on my alarm (I'm usually up before it goes off) and I weigh 119 pounds.

Mentally, severe sleep deprivation can make us irrational, uncoordinated and slow-witted, but unaware of our impairment. Studies have shown sleepy people at the wheel have as many accidents as drug-impaired drivers. While you sleep, your brain cleverly works on the problems of the day, helping you make better decisions. Scientists know they can study the facts of a problem and "sleep on it," knowing that their brains will keep piecing together the facts of a puzzle long into the night. Some people keep pencils and notepads next to their bed to write down any late-night ideas. Sometimes in the morning on the floor next to their beds, they find the solutions they are looking for.

Emotionally, your dreams are your personal vision of heaven and your nightmares are your personal vision of hell. You may be stuffing down feelings, but they will come out somehow. Whenever I dream about not being able to close the door on my bathroom, that's a signal for me to get some time and space for myself. And I do it.

Spiritually, your dreams help you make sense of the world. Native peoples, who often have the least in material goods, use their dreams as guides for their daily lives. I read an interview with a tribe member whose most prized possession was his spear. His biggest fear was for the young people and that "They got no dreamin'." In other words, he saw that people were emphasizing their physical world and becoming strangers to their spiritual side.

Get your required amount of sleep. Only you can decide how much you need. Go to bed at a set time for a few days and see what time you wake up without an alarm. How many hours do you sleep in that time? Use it as your guideline. By eating well, exercising and getting your beauty sleep, you will have reserves for when it's truly necessary to skimp on sleep – like when that big project is due, a family emergency occurs or when you're on that fun vacation. Sleep deprivation is a tried and true method of torture. Don't do it to yourself.

While you are thinking about it, fill in some of the blanks below, then think about ways you can fill your own needs.

I need _____ in my life.

1.

2.

3.

4.

5.

I need **more** _____ in my life.

1.

2.

3.

4.

5.

I need **less** _____ in my life.

1.

2.

3.

4.

5.

Chapter 7

Questions to Ask

A healthy person is one who can look at situations and problems and, by analyzing their choices and following them through, achieve the best possible result. They set their own autopilots, so their thoughts and activities help them reach their goals rather than hold them back.

I can't tell you what choices to make, but I can give you questions to answer. Your answers will clue you in on what to look for when choices come your way. Life isn't perfect; it's a constant struggle. It has a way of smacking you when you say, "I'm not going to let that happen anymore," because, invariably, it does. I think it's best to say to yourself, "If *that* ever happens again, I'll be able to deal." And do it.

If you want to work on your life, it's important to ask, "Who sets my autopilot? Why do I do the things that I do?"

What is Your Party for One?

Are you happy with yourself when you're by yourself? You can tell a lot about your self-esteem by the party you throw for yourself. If your alone time is *always* spent cleaning the house or doing the laundry, look for ways to treat yourself better. What do you do when you don't have to answer to anyone? Your party for one ought to include something physical, and shopping doesn't count. Ideally, it should include something mentally stimulating you can talk about later, so that means the treadmill is out, too. Is it something someone else might want to join you in? How can you attract good company if you can't have fun by yourself? I like to do all kinds of things by myself. My party for one is often a bike ride or a long walk or a hike. I'll take myself out to lunch or to an art gallery or to South America. Sure, I like to do things with others, but I don't let their schedules affect how I treat myself. It's what I do for me.

What is your Art Form?

When I was a make-up artist, I knew that my art would go down the drain each night, but believe me, I still took a huge amount of pleasure in my work. The fact that it was only temporary didn't make it any less important.

I lived for the moment to see a woman look into the mirror and have her eyes light up with satisfaction, even if it was just for a split second. They knew they were beautiful and I got satisfaction in knowing I helped them see that beauty.

Your art form can be anything you want it to be, but *it must be yours alone.* It will connect you to the rest of humanity, and that is worthwhile for it's own sake. Only humans express themselves through art. From the pre-historic cave paintings in France to modern media, art means that we have been here and we have made a difference.

Artists become keepers of rituals and connections to humanity by helping people see things they might otherwise miss. As a make up artist and clothing sales person, I think I helped women see the beauty in themselves. It didn't matter to me if my art was going down the drain or in the hamper that night. It did what it needed to do.

Your art form could be a perfectly pressed collar, a presentation worthy of repeating, or a fine meal. Anything you feel you do well qualifies. Here is an example:

There is a very large snail that is a delicacy in southern waters called a conch (pronounced "conk"). When it is cooked properly, it is heavenly. I can remember almost every time I've eaten it and the sunset that went along with it. It has to be lovingly tenderized with vinegars or pounded within an eighth of an inch with a hammer. If it's cooked wrong, it's like an old shoe.

An old man I've seen on my trips in the Bahamas always appears shirtless and shoeless, sitting in a very old boat. He dives for conch during the day and in the late afternoons, he cleans them to sell. Around 3 p.m. each afternoon, he'll shout "Showtime!" while cleaning conch as people gather to buy the conch meat and see his show. He says that cleaning conch is the only thing he does well, but I think that's all he needs to do. It's his art form and he has perfected it.

At one point in my college career, I believed that one should exclusively work on ones deficiencies. I let *all* my time be taken up by things I wasn't good at and didn't like to do. I took classes in subjects I struggled with and I did this on purpose. I figured that if I could do well in subjects I wasn't good at, all the rest would take care of itself. I was totally wrong – and totally miserable. I was not doing *any* of my art forms: the things I loved and enjoyed. Of course, you have to do things you don't like in life, but at some point, you have to do what you are good at and enjoy on a regular basis. I know from personal experience that if you don't make time to enjoy your art forms, you will be miserable and drag down everyone around you, too.

Everyone should have an their art form that they choose for themselves. The road is there – find it for yourself.

Others' Art Forms

One thing I don't do as an art form is to conform to others' art forms. Anyone who has ever picked up a magazine and wished they looked like the model on the cover should understand the following:

Actors and models are packaged entertainment products, just like books and DVD's. Their images and actions are carefully choreographed so that you will buy them. Images in popular culture are works of art for the person who created them: *their* art form. They are no more representative of real life than a Monet painting. The people who create these images usually have no interest in females, anyway. Don't try to conform to their representations. I like to look at fashion magazines to get ideas about fun things that I want to *do* or clothes to *wear*, not what I should *be*.

Remember when we talked about choosing your art form? Your art form should be in your *life* and not in your *appearance*.

Images in magazines and movies are a moment in time. They are air brushed and digitally altered until the real life model bears no resemblance to it. Really, do you think models in cosmetic ads have no pores? No one is getting plastic surgery to look like a Picasso or Dali painting – advertisements shouldn't be any different. It drives me crazy that many women try to make themselves into living images of someone else's fantasy. What's worse is that perfectly straight men will buy into this fantasy and think that's what a woman "should" look like.

When I get dolled up as the living image of someone's fantasy girl, it's either *my* fantasy or that of someone I know. I love to play the glamour girl game once in a while, but that's all it is for me: a fun game. When it stops being fun, I stop the game. You can only lose when the glamour game isn't a game anymore. Be careful when the game becomes your life – you can end up like the high school quarterback who threw the winning touchdown in 1972. If how you looked at 27 is the highest point of your life – well, what have you got to look forward to? You have to put your eye on another prize.

What's in Your Lemonade Stand?

As kids, we set up lemonade stands by the side of the road to earn money. It was fun. We made money. It's the American way. Each time you stop to buy a cup you see the thrill on the faces of those kids. But somewhere along the way, in the pressure to make money, the fun got lost. Most people are miserable in their jobs. It doesn't have to be that way.

In days past, people knew if they worked for a company for 20 or 30 years, a pension check would arrive in the mailbox every month until the day they died. The phrase was "job security," and it is unfamiliar to today's workers.

Our economy has changed dramatically in the past few years, and the days of employer/employee loyalty will probably never return. The main contributor for this change is "switching costs." In years past, customers who needed goods and services found it very difficult to switch from one supplier to another. Now, the ease at which customers can make their choices is almost ridiculous. Low switching costs have decimated job security. I believe that part of the huge amount of stress that people feel in their lives is not knowing whether or not they will have a job in five years or even five months.

In the mortgage business, people used their local banker for everything from a savings account to a car loan to a mortgage. The banker could charge whatever he wanted and the customer would take it or leave it. If the customer wanted to shop around, it was a time consuming ordeal. Then brokers became the preferred source for mortgage money. The customer visited a broker who would shop for rates at different lenders. Now, on the Internet, people can go to businesses that present several brokers to each customer. Over time, different types of businesses have become "the source" for mortgage money. This business evolution has happened for every type of business, but it now happens faster and faster with both good and bad consequences.

To keep from being overwhelmed, think about what service you can offer your employers or customers that they would find hard to get anywhere else. What can you add to your lemonade stand? It may be as simple as a warm greeting and a smile. There is a lot of money in the world and it ebbs and flows like the tides. It may take some thinking on your part, but you can ride the wave if you find the way.

In my lemonade stand, there are three simple things that have helped me with my own career success. First, I like to look at a job and see if there is one little thing I could do to make it better. I go the extra "inch." In the minds of others it is measured as a mile, and they always admire the extra effort.

Second, I review and follow up. Few people do this with any regularity – if you do, it will put you on top. When everyone else is frazzled and playing catch-up, take time to review what it is you need to do for people. Set some time aside once a week – two hours is plenty – and go through your files or contacts. Think about whom you need to communicate with to make sure "everything is on track." It takes nine times longer to fix a mistake than to do it correctly in the first place. Some simple checks will allow you to catch problems before they happen and you'll be way ahead of the game.

Finally, no matter how mundane the job is, strive to do it better. When I worked at the clothing store, I could have just put away the clothes, but the ladies would tell me where they were going and I would dress them for the occasion. I spent time studying the new fashions and putting them together with accessories: it was an art form for me. I wouldn't let them leave unless they looked *good*.

Later, they would come back, tell me the outfit I had found for them was perfect and now they needed one for *another* occasion. I was only 17 years old. I had never been to these fancy places, but I stayed on top of fashions, did my best and made a lot of money. Even now, I have confidence to try new things because I can say to myself: "If it doesn't work out, I can go back to selling dresses."

Life *will* give you lemons. Have a few lemonade recipes. A little special attention can make the difference between a job and a career. None of my suggestions take more than a few minutes a day, but for me, they have made the difference between stress and confidence, failure and success.

What do you Fear?

Without fear, there is no courage. Fears are just as personal as hungers and are just as often denied. People who profess to have no fear aren't in touch with their humanity. Machines have no fear.

Fear is a genuinely helpful emotion. It helps you recognize when things go wrong. Unfortunately, those who may not have your best interests at heart constantly manipulate your fears. You may fear dying or having no money or love or "ring around the collar."

When you face your fear, you stop running. The energy used to avoid a problem is now spent solving the problem. If you can look your fear in the eye and say, "Bring it on!," then you will be on your way to achieving the self-esteem you deserve. Sometimes you have to be at the end of a dead-end tunnel to force yourself to turn around, but it's at that point you start a new game and set the rules yourself.

Let your fear motivate you. When things are out of control, you must put *your* force behind a change. But you don't have to do it alone. Look to see what choices you have to leverage your resources. Choice is leverage and leverage moves the world.

What is your Everest?

Your Everest is whatever preoccupies your mind. I have had a whole mountain range of Everest's to conquer. Lousy jobs, fear of failure, bad relationships, no money – you name it, it has been thrown my way. But, my reaction to stress has always been to get to the root of the problem and to strengthen myself in the process.

An Everest prevents you from living in the current moment. Rather, you obsess about the past and worry about the future. It is a problem you must overcome, because if you deal with these concerns in an unreal time, be it the past or the future, nothing will ever change. The past and an inability to live in the present will prevent you from achieving your goals for the future. And often, we do everything we can to avoid difficult situations and people. Think about why television is so popular. It allows you to be entertained while your mind is preoccupied with other problems. TV allows you to fool yourself into believing that all your problems will be resolved before the next commercial break. Wouldn't that be wonderful?

Unfortunately, if you are not looking at your Everest directly, facing your situation squarely, you will never rise above it. You need to know how high is the climb. You need to know what gear you need, and how you can train for it. You need to know on whom you can depend to guide you. Edmund Hillary, the first man to conquer the real Mount Everest in 1953, would still be at the bottom if it weren't for Tenzing Norgay, his Sherpa guide. You need to know how long it will take and how you will know when you've reached the summit. It might take the rest of your life, but the rest of your life is what you've got. And if you don't climb it, what will you have? You'll have the same (or bigger) problem, but less time to deal with it. And although reaching the top may seem insurmountable, you can break your problem down into manageable steps. You can't climb a mountain in a day, but you can take one step at a time.

Let's say you hate your job. You could stay and be miserable, or try to find a solution to your problem. One common solution is returning to school to obtain the skills necessary to find a new position. You might hesitate about returning to school because you are already imagining yourself cramming for finals. This fear will paralyze you before you even begin.

Take it one small step at a time. One day, stop by a college and pick up a catalog. Another day, pick it up and look at it. It won't burn a hole in your hands. Look at the class descriptions and see if there is something that interests you. If there is, get an application. Fill out the first line, then the second and so on until you are done. So what if it takes a week or two? You are still making those first steps to climb to the top of that problem.

Another common stumbling block is money. Maybe you don't have money for tuition and books. Don't let that stop you; there are plenty of people with money who want to help others *who deserve it*. Start with your boss or the financial aid office at the school. Search online for grants or scholarships. Companies receive tax breaks for paying employees' tuition (even though you don't) and schools are dedicated to filling every seat in their classrooms. Other concerns include time and good childcare: you need to recognize how much time you will need and when you will need it to achieve your goals. But, look around. There are plenty of people in the same situation that can help you if you ask. For years, I swapped weekly childcare with other moms. The kids get to play together and we got some time for our own pursuits.

I find that if I face a problem squarely and analyze it directly, I am able to recognize the people in my life who can help me on the journey. Don't be dismayed if you don't currently have a network of friends who fit the bill. I am amazed by the people I meet in "chance" situations who have helped me accomplish my goals. Shakespeare said, "All the world's a stage," and sometimes it seems that these people who appear in my life have been waiting backstage until some director sends them out when I need them most.

For example, I was putting together a reading program at my daughter's school and the person I knew who could help me the most was not someone I would run into on an ordinary day. But, we met up by chance and discussed it. When I told her that I was thinking of her and needed her help, she said, "Well then, you just conjured me up!" And you know, I probably did. Sometimes I don't recognize these people at first, but they seem to come back again and again to inspire or help me.

Sometimes I just sit with a blank piece of paper and a pen at a table and think about where I want to be and the problems I want to overcome. This eliminates distractions and helps me evaluate what I have to work with and what I need. Then I make my list and look around. You can recognize this process from the way I choose my foods and the way I pick my clothes. I use it all the time, especially with things that are important to me.

The world is a generous place that can provide you with everything you need to live a good and satisfying life. Sometimes we need to go out and find the things to meet our needs and not wait until they come to us.

Sometimes it is OK to be Scarlett O'Hara and think about your problems tomorrow. Just make sure tomorrow comes. In the meantime, deliberately let your sadness or fear or anger wash over you. Let it tell you what you need to know. Don't run from it, otherwise you will be running for the rest of your life. When times seem to be at their worst for me, I stop and face my problems. Believe me, one of the most powerful feelings is knowing you can conquer the obstacles in your way.

When you go climbing, ropes and walkways help guide you and keep you safe. Did you ever wonder who put those safety ropes in place? Those people have the skills, expertise and courage that novice climbers and hikers don't have and probably couldn't get. This example can be carried across many other situations. When you are climbing your Everest, remember that whatever you are facing now, others have gone before you and triumphed. Watch and learn from them. Someone, somewhere can help you deal with what you are facing now. You never know, it could be this book you are holding right now. And finally, don't think about falling: think about the view when you get there.

What is your Refuge?

Or what would you like your refuge to be? Your refuge is where you go to restore *all* forms of your health. You might need more than one. Is it the bathtub or under a tree? Is it out on the water or with a group of friends? You need to set up a refuge or two for regular use.

I keep both solitary and group pursuits as my refuges. Most of them don't call for eating. Sewing, for example, is one of my favorite and most easily accessible mental refuges. If I were chowing down on Cheetos while I worked, I would ruin my art. Gardening is a terrific physical refuge. You can eat the fruits of your labor, but that's only after you clean up. When you scuba dive, you can't even talk, much less eat, and it restores me in every way.

I also take spiritual refuge in helping those in need. I've been tutoring once every other week for years and I have belonged to groups who helped in major ways like raising funds to buy electric wheelchairs and study materials for reading programs.

In the first chapter, I asked you to think about what you were *really* hungry for. Feed those hungers with your refuges instead of food.

What is in Your Spiritual Medicine Cabinet?

You have to have all of you engaged to live a full life. This means valuing all of you: not just your physical side, but your mental, emotional and spiritual sides as well. Spiritually healthy people know they will hurt at one time or another. They are masters at marshalling the resources that will help them overcome the pain. Did you toss out all your knives the first time you got a cut? No, you went for a Band-Aid and ointment.

You have resources for physical pain, but you need resources for mental, emotional and spiritual pain, too. These resources are friends you can talk to, books you can read, church or synagogue congregations, or other groups with whom you can commiserate. These resources can help you come to terms with the feelings you are dealing with. Sometimes everything *won't* be all right, but you can still find your place in the world.

Many people look to pop culture for gods and goddesses to use as guides and to emulate. But, you can look at hundreds of different religions throughout time to find your "invisible means of support." You may have to look outside of your own religion if you aren't gaining the inspiration and motivation you need. The Greeks and Romans had wonderful gods and goddesses that helped them find their place in the universe. Many western institutions were invented within these societies. Hindu and Buddhist gods and goddesses also inspire us. Saraswati is the Hindu goddess of knowledge and the arts. Buddhist Bodhisattvas, both male and female, are examples and teachers of great compassion. White Tara is a renowned goddess of strength and generosity. Men who practice western religions might not understand, but it does a lot for a woman's self-esteem to be able to say. "Wow, she's incredible and *I'm just like her!*" Native American, African and other religions that teach the human connection to divine power through the earth are worth a closer look too.

What is your Third Option?

Many people look at situations as either/or propositions. You can have one thing – or another. One is wrong and one is right. One is a winner and one is a loser. It's black, or it's white. That is not always true. People who only see black or white have sensory deprivation. Almost every situation has a shade of gray. I always look for the third option. Some people call it a "win-win" situation where everyone's needs are met. It's in there somewhere and I find the search for it very satisfying.

For example, if the boss asks if you can stay after quitting time, you can say "Yes" and get picked on every time, or you can say "no" and not be a "team player." Setting limits or conditions is the reason for looking for your third option. Your third option can be, "Yes. I can stay until 6." By putting a condition on your work relationship, everyone is a winner. The boss gets the extra work done; you miss the traffic and get "team player" status. If you say "yes," work 'til nine and miss your dinner plans: you are filled with resentment and are heading for a life that is permanently out of balance.

Another example: I like to go to ballet performances and when my husband lost his job, my obvious choices were to continue going and spend money we didn't have, or stop going altogether and lose a part of myself. I couldn't do either. But after a while I realized I could *volunteer* to help the company in a number of different ways. To make a long story short: I saw *every* performance from *very* expensive seats.

Resetting your Autopilot

What are the motivations of the people who are passing on their beliefs to you? Why do you believe them? What have the answers to these questions told you about yourself? Can you look back and understand where some of your beliefs and actions come from? And can you change them to serve you?

You can find spiritual health by facing the trials of your Everest and by feeling the power that comes when you overcome your obstacles. You can find your place in the world through your art. Find your art and perform it – it will lead you to the balance and beauty that lies within you.

When you turn your thoughts toward your problems and take small steps in that direction, the keys to solving your problems seem to appear before your eyes. This is not magic. It happens because you are widening your radar screen. We can't change the river, we can only steer the currents. You can row against the current or let it take you where you want to go. Your future comes from your mind. The choices you make either consciously or unconsciously determine the course of your life. It's *your* choice. Make it.

Chapter 8

Food *is* Love, Food *is* Life

If food chemists could synthesize a pill that could give people all the nutrition they need at one gulp – it would never sell. We love our food. We love the taste of it, the feel of it and the idea of it too much to give it up. As much trouble as food is for us, it is worth it. It means so much more to us than what is on the plate in front of us.

Life, love and food go together. Your life should be arranged around the things you love. Your life also depends on the food you eat. You should have the foods you love arranged in your life so that, like good friends who support you, they are there when you need them. Your food should be a source of strength, not a weakness.

As the cliché "you are what you eat," says: you really *are* what you eat. How can you be anything else? Therefore, you have to eat what you are. You are proteins and vitamins and fats and minerals and water. You have to eat these things on a daily basis or your earthly incarnation will cease to exist. All that will be left is the memory of what you have accomplished.

Is there any kind of gathering that doesn't involve food? Family gatherings and celebrations revolve around the meal. But the funny thing is, every gathering may involve food, but it's not *about* the food. It's about the relationships you have with the people with whom you share food.

If food is love, then *offer* your love to yourself and others. Don't force it on anyone, but offer. Forcing people to eat what they don't want and restricting what they do will backfire. I can only tell you what goes on in my own family, but we eat a lot of apples and broccoli, and the chocolate Easter bunnies on the snack shelf get thrown away some time in July.

Food is Communication

Food is communication. We know how others feel about us by the food they provide. It is body language of the most basic sort. Our very first inkling of love comes from the food we are nourished with. It gives us life and along with it, love.

People express their love through food. For many, cooking for loved ones is a source of pride. I think that everyone should have a dish they are proud of and can lovingly share with others in their lives. Have you ever seen the light in a child's eyes when they've made breakfast in bed for their parents? You don't have to be a master cook, but the ability to nourish oneself and others is a pleasure I think one should not live without.

A lot of women naturally gravitate to the kitchen. Mothers give life (with help from fathers, of course) and continue in that role, by nourishing themselves and their families. It makes sense that the one who gives life would continue as the food giver, but why should women have that honor all to themselves? I can't think of a better way for the rest of the family to feel a sense of belonging than to have everyone oooohh and ahhh over something they have prepared themselves.

Food is Feelings

How you feel about food can influence your life for better or for worse. The quality of your children's lives is also affected by your eating habits, the examples you set and the rules you make. You can make the eating experience pleasurable or painful for everybody in your family.

One of my rules for food preparation is that everybody helps out in the kitchen. Like any manager, it is my job to see that we have a pleasant atmosphere, but everybody pitches in. I have kids, especially, help with the vegetable preparation. Even the smallest child can help with the washing. They love to splash around in a sink full of water. And they actually eat a larger variety of foods because they are already familiar with them. I still remember when my three-year-old in the baby carrier on the grocery cart said, "Don't forget the broccoli, Mom." The other produce customers almost fell over.

Late one afternoon, my daughter's friend came over. Her mother spent quite some time telling me exactly what her daughter would and wouldn't eat for dinner. When we divvied up the food preparation, her job was to fix the snow peas – washing them and pulling off the strings. I stir-fried them in a little oil and gave her a wooden spoon so she could "cook," too. She ate a whole plateful of them and now her mom makes them for her all the time. This was a child that supposedly would eat nothing but potatoes.

Another time, I had a houseful of children while I was cooking dinner, and my three-year-old nephew asked if he could help out by cutting the green beans. I was a little hesitant, so I asked him if he would show me how he cut. His technique was flawless: he had a firm grip on the (small) knife and held his thumb in while he cupped the food to hold it. I was incredulous, so I said to him, "Christopher! You are only three years old and your mother lets you cut with a *sharp* knife??!!" He replied, "No, she doesn't. But I'm going to tell her that YOU did." Needless to say, I found another job for him, but I was happy that he had an interest in good food even at that young age.

My second rule is that everyone can have more. I serve small portions and let everyone know that if they finish, they can get a second helping. This has the effect of slowing down the eating experience so that it is more enjoyable and fulfilling. Guests at my table have to really think about whether or not they want that second helping instead of mindlessly finishing everything they see on their plate.

My last rule is that everyone has to have a little bit of everything on the plate. I put two bites worth of every dish on each child's plate. It takes between three and seven exposures to a new food to get someone to try it. You should see the looks I get when I tell kids, "You don't have to eat it, but you have to look at it." How can kids try a new food if it is not *offered* to them? And how can they hate something when they are not forced to eat it?

I don't have problems with "picky eaters," and it's an easy way to get people to try more foods. One of the easiest ways to be healthy is to eat a wide variety of foods. If the small servings go in the garbage, it's a small sacrifice to make for good nutrition. I would rather sacrifice a little food than my family's health and enjoyment.

One easy way to show kids what is good food and what isn't is to give it the hamster test. Our hamster will eat healthy foods like carrots and bananas, but will turn her nose up at over-processed foods, like candy and chips. I figure that if the hamster likes it, it has to be good – and the children follow her good example.

Where Do You Live?

Ou habite vous? That's French for "Where do you live?" It's no coincidence the English word for habit is the French word for live. Your habits *are* your life. For some of us, our habits are the choices we make day after day. For many of us, our habits consist of what is easiest to do in a stressed-out world. Many people don't take the time to make conscious decisions on even the most basic necessities. We just go with the flow and hope for the best.

Don't believe in the fallacy that you are born with the body you have and there is nothing you can do about it. You have the body you deserve. If you eat well and are active, you are in much better shape than your relatives who don't. The good news is you can start to make better choices, *today*.

I'm a military brat, so my family traveled everywhere when I was young. I still have major wanderlust. Traveling has helped me understand other cultures and their attitudes toward food. Most often, their attitudes are much healthier than ours. Nobody eats more processed food than Americans. Many of us can go for weeks without eating a single food in its natural state. The only thing with a label that a lot of Europeans ingest is wine.

Think about it: Do you ever see an advertisement for a green pepper? Is your local farmer parading around in sexy clothes, tantalizing you with a lovely salad? No way! Those hard working people are up to their ankles in mud to make sure we (and most of the rest of the world) are getting enough to eat. A modern farmer can get 10 times as much food from an acre of land than could his or her great-grandparents.

Advertising is what the other guys, the "processors" use to get products to the top of your mind. They want their products to be "top of mind" – the first thing we think about when we get a craving. This takes many, many repetitions, until the message is drilled into peoples' heads. The concept is similar to intensive training or brain washing. And it costs a lot of money. The only food products that make enough profit to advertise over and over are processed foods. I'm not saying we shouldn't eat processed food, but you weren't meant to live on a diet of cold cuts and potato chips, no matter what that hotdog guy says.

It is no coincidence that pizza commercials appear during the 5 o'clock news. The pizza delivery chains know you just got home from work *both* tired and in a panic that that you have to put together a meal for yourself and your family or guests. They offer a great suggestion: "One call and dinner is at the door." And it's true. Being able to speed dial those seven numbers and have nature's perfect food come to your doorstep in less than an hour is the Eighth Wonder of the World, as far as I'm concerned. The trouble is that it does nothing to help you eat a variety of food. There is another way.

Planning vs. Scheduling, Part I

A lot of people get planning and scheduling confused. Planning is looking to see where or what *you want to be* and then looking at *where you are now*. Figuring what steps you need to take to get from one to the other may seem like the hard part. Scheduling is figuring out *when* you are going to do these things. I find following through with the scheduling is the hard part. Planning means nothing without scheduling, and scheduling means nothing without planning. If you do one without the other, you have wasted your time.

Menu Planning

Menu planning for me is keeping a list of food that is in the deep recesses of my freezer and pantries that I can make with the fresh foods I buy on a weekly basis. All I need to do is glance at my list to schedule a meal when I need one. <u>Chapter 9</u> shows you the whole process, but the following illustrates how it affects your *life*.

The Payoff

Early evenings are a battleground in a lot of families. People come home to find refuge from the stresses of their day and find more stressors waiting to pounce on them at home. Dads find their easy chairs and remotes; kids escape to their rooms, and moms start the second shift. These are habits that become people's lives. Is this what you really want?

You have to fight this habit like no other battle you have ever fought. But the key is to fight the stress – not each other. I know you can't do this every night, but once in a while, for 30 minutes, try a new strategy. I find that this works for me.

Fight the temptation to turn on the evening news. You have enough horror stories from your own day without getting caught up in somebody else's tragedy. The TV is an escape from your own stress: if you are running from your problems, they won't be solved.

If you can't live without the news, record it for later. If the stories concern you, then you know more than the reporters do already. The silence will be hard to take. Instead, turn on some soothing music.

Music really can soothe a savage beast. My daughter bought me an hour-long spa CD that is permanently in a CD player. It has all the sounds I love, like crashing waves and violins. When things get out of hand around here, even she will press the play button. I also have a radio preset to the smooth jazz station.

Go into the kitchen, the heart of your home. Collect your thoughts for five minutes and plan the next hour. Mentally divide up mealtime duties. You already have what you need. There is preparation, presentation, and then more preparation.

Insist the kids turn off whatever electronic device they are using and join you there. Let them bring their homework or something else of interest to them. Tell then specifically that you want to spend time with them. It will be music to their ears, even if they don't acknowledge it. Fight the temptation to let those surly brats stew in their rooms. Believe me, the time when they need you the most is when they are at their worst.

Exchange back or neck rubs. Stress seems to manifest itself in these two areas and a two-minute rub can relieve it better than a shakerful of martinis. Believe it or not, your kids really want your (positive) attention and want to be with you. Even two-year-olds enjoy running wheeled massagers on their parents.

After a few quiet moments, assign jobs to your helpers. The same two-year-old loves washing lettuce and green beans in a sink full of water. I keep plastic cups and napkins in a low cabinet so everybody can take part in setting the table.

Prepare your meal together and present it lovingly. I will tell you how I manage from the moment I begin until the final clean up in <u>Chapter 12</u>, <u>The Skinny Girl Cooks</u>. Afterward, clean up the mess together. *Everyone* has to at least bring his or her dishes to the sink. When the kitchen is clean, take five minutes to think about what you'll serve for your next meal. When the time comes, you won't be faced with a sink full of dishes and you will be ready to prepare what you *want* to eat instead of stressing about it.

Then, take the dog (or yourself) for a walk to clear your head for the next challenge.

Let the evening meal become a feast for all five senses: sight, hearing, touch, taste and smell. Try to put on this feast as often as you can. When you try to change your family's direction, they may fight you tooth and nail. Some people hate change, even if it is for the better. But I find that things go much more smoothly when we take some time to unwind together every day. You might find that your family is actually eager to join you in these rituals. I know I hurry home if there's a good meal and a back rub waiting for me.

In the next section, I'll tell you all about S.W.A.T. cooking and how you can make meal preparation as easy as possible. Also in <u>Chapter 12</u>, I'll tell you how to set up your kitchen so you can get the maximum benefit from a small space. You really can fix a good meal more easily, more cheaply and most important, more enjoyably than ordering take out every night.

S.W.A.T. Cooking

There are times in your life when you can see stress coming right toward you. If you're an accountant, you can see April 15th on the calendar. If you are a student, final exams come up with regularity. New parents prepare for a due date. Old parents prepare for the holidays. Everyone has an end of the month or end of the year due date, or a big project to deliver to a very picky client.

Then there are the times when stress pops up unexpectedly. A loved one is injured in an accident, or someone gets sick and needs your help. Or that big opportunity you've been waiting for all your life comes along and you have just a small window of time to seize it. Both good and bad, there are as many situations that need your undivided attention as there are people in your life. And in these stressful situations, you still need to eat. If you are going to eat well, you need to have a plan for these times.

S.W.A.T. stands for Special Weapons And Tactics. Most people identify S.W.A.T. teams with military troops or rescue squads that help out in stressful situations when life and limb are on the line. Sometimes you get in a stressful situation where *your* life is on the line. It may not be that you are going to lose it, but the *quality* of your life, for better or worse, will be affected by how you act under stress, right now. You can triumph, or you can go down.

One quiet afternoon very soon, go through your recipes and make a list of 10 meals that you can fix quickly and easily. Make sure that your ingredients include foods that have vitamins and minerals that you are not getting from your multi-vitamin. See <u>Chapter 10</u>, <u>Eating Right by Sight</u>, and the appendix for help. This is more difficult than it sounds. Divide these up into two groups of five. Make copies of each recipe (*you* may have them memorized, but others may not) and a grocery list for each group of meals.

You now have two weeks of grocery lists and recipes planned ahead of time. Stash these in a convenient place for use when you really need them. Sometimes I alternate each group of recipes every other week for several months and no one notices. You can't remember what it was you ate a week ago Tuesday and neither can your family. This also works great because you can then give your grocery list or recipes to someone who wants to be of help during your trying time. There is no fumbling through cookbooks, and you already know that the food will be both tasty and healthful. The help you need now meets the S.M.A.R.T. parameters we discussed in the <u>Chapter 6</u> and you will find it so much easier to obtain.

What Do You Know?

What do you know about the food you are going to need tomorrow? If you just now started thinking about today's meals, you are too late. I need something for three meals a day, something to sip on, something to snack on, and something to eat on the run.

I pick these out ahead of time. I also keep a whole shelf in my refrigerator for what I call "grab and stuff." The concept is just like it sounds – you grab it and you stuff it in your mouth. On my "grab and stuff" shelf are grapes, strawberries, yogurt, string cheese and bottled water. *Behind* them is the chocolate. They are not substitutes for my meals, but I don't like to leave the house hungry. I do this because I want to keep my energy up and I can't think clearly when I'm hungry. And although I could skip the "grab and stuff" and head to the candy aisle or the bakery, I'd rather have foods that do things *for* me, not *to* me. I would eat a whole box of pastry if you put it in front of me and I was hungry enough, but it's not something that happens because I make a decision to eat well – and before I leave the house.

You *know* you are going to get hungry a few times a day. Make your decisions ahead of time. Eat breakfast! Know what you are going to have for your midmorning snack instead of planning *nothing*. If you plan *nothing,* then what's going to happen when you do get hungry? You'll take whatever is there. You won't lose weight by not eating. Your body will find a way to compensate. Your metabolism will slow, or you'll binge and be angry with yourself, or you will die from starvation. In any case, *you* lose and so does everybody else.

If you still don't believe the quality of your food affects the quality of your life, maybe the next story will help.

I went to elementary school with a pretty girl named Karen. I used to sit next to her at lunch. One day she started to bring huge amounts of food to lunch every day and ate every bite. I asked her why. She answered that she wanted to be at her "perfect weight." She was *eleven* years old. Not knowing or caring what that meant, I asked her about it anyway. She told me that she had seen a height and weight table and that her weight was too low for her height.

The years went by and we lost touch in middle school. In high school, Karen and I had the same lunch period and started sitting together at lunch again. This time however, all she brought to eat were hard-boiled eggs and carrot sticks. She told me that she had gained way too much weight and now she was trying to lose it. It was horrible to watch her, day after day, choking down that awful lunch and not looking up at me or anybody else.

Pretty soon there were parties and other social occasions opening up for my classmates and I. We went horseback riding and water-skiing. We played tennis in the park. We biked over to each other's houses. We went out for cheering squads and track. But Karen never went. When my other friends and I chattered away, chowing down on pizza or burgers and fries at lunch, she would sit by herself, with her carrot sticks and hard-boiled eggs, miserably trying to fit into that perfect slot on the height and weight chart. I never kept in touch with her after high school. I still feel sorry for her.

There are thousands of people like Karen out there, asking themselves if they are too fat instead of what kind of great adventure they can have today. They are shortchanging themselves and the world around them because the gifts they have to offer are being held hostage in a body trying to obtain the "perfect weight." I hate to say it, but I didn't care about my perfect weight then and I don't care now. My perfect weight is what I am. Food is my fuel to stay strong and healthy. If it gives me enough energy to drag myself out of bed and stand on two legs – well then, it's going to be a great day!

I shudder to think what my life would have been like if I had asked to see that stupid chart.

Food is Community

You can use food to express your love to people other than your family and friends. There is a special feeling you get when you know that your actions will make a real difference in a person's life: like the world is a better place because you passed this way. You can't get that feeling at the bottom of a gallon of ice cream. Here's an example:

One year I gave a "White Christmas" to a single mom and her two kids who were on welfare. I went to the local warehouse store and bought everything white that I could find. A fifty-pound sack of rice, a fifty-pound sack of flour, a twenty-pound sack of sugar, salt, shampoo, toothpaste, soap, paper towels, toilet paper, facial tissue. All of it cost less than $100.

I sent cards to four friends to whom I would have otherwise sent a $25 knick-knack to let them know what they had done for this lady. It cost me nothing. My friends were thrilled. She was thrilled. I was thrilled and found it *very* satisfying. It took pressure off of her – welfare doesn't cover basic necessities like soap, shampoo and toothpaste – the very things one needs to get a job. She had other help, of course, and has worked extremely hard. Now, she's a supervisor at her company and her kids are on the honor roll at their school. That's real help that *you* can do, too.

If you don't know what to do yourself, call a church, homeless shelter or school. The person who answers the phone can direct your help (money, goods, time or energy) to someone who really needs it. That one phone call can satisfy a lot of needs that a whole bag of cookies would never touch. If you want to obsess about food, your obsession should be about getting food to people who don't have enough. There is always something you can do to help others and it doesn't always take money.

Keep Trying

A word about failure: Do you remember when you were learning to walk? Of course you don't – it was too painful and we block those things out. Watch a baby try it. They pull themselves up a little and they fall down. Sometimes they cry, but after a while they try again. Do you really think you tried it once and said to yourself, "This is too hard! I give up!" No, you kept at it so you aren't still scooting yourself across your mother's kitchen floor.

You may find some of the strategies in this book to be awkward – or too challenging – at first, but don't give up. The rewards are tremendous when you succeed. Living *well* is the best. It's not living skinny or rich.

Chapter 9

A Look At Other Cultures

We can see where we get our habits when we look at other cultures around the world and in our own past. Some of them worked very well in a different place and time. But, here we are in *this* place, and *this* time, and it seems like *everyone* is unhappy with his or her weight.

Ancient Cultures

Let's think about where our "knowledge" of food comes from. Food is light energy from the sun. No wonder the sun was worshipped as a god by many ancient cultures. To them, life itself was given by the sun. Planets too far from the sun are cold and dead.

Many holidays, like Halloween and Easter, have their roots in traditions and rituals that our ancient ancestors practiced because they believed they would bring the sun back from wherever it went in the cold and dark of wintertime.

In ancient Europe, people believed the earth died every fall and was "reborn" in the spring. The scary images of Halloween were an attempt by people to understand what was about to happen in their world. All they knew was that the sun would shine less and less each day. The leaves would fall from every tree except the evergreens, which would eventually be celebrated as the only living thing left in winter. The animals would leave to hibernate. The ground froze and was covered with snow. Streams iced over. There would be no readily available food or water. To them, the world, and everything in it, was dying.

Think about how *you* would feel if you went into the kitchen and there was no water from the tap and no food in the cupboards? Pretty desperate?

Even in places with mild winters, such as Florida, some situations can put you right back in the Middle Ages. The first thing hurricane preparedness information sources tell you is to fill the tub with drinking water after rinsing it out with bleach, and to stock up on canned goods and a manual can opener, as well as a flashlight and a lot of batteries. People can get pretty desperate in the dark with no food or water.

Many superstitions evolved in an attempt to bring back the sun and its life-giving food and water. Then, as if by magic, the sun would move closer and stay for hours more each day. Trees and plants sprouted and streams thawed. Animals came out of hiding and there was food for everyone.

So, food was, therefore, a gift from god. Ancient cultures spent so much of their daily lives in pursuit of enough to eat that it was blasphemous to waste such a gift. Many of us carry on that tradition by saying a prayer of thanks before we eat our meals. Some of us carry it even further by considering not finishing everything on the plate to be an insult to the God who delivered it. But, come on now! We have to get over that. The pizza guy isn't God!

Up until about 100 years ago (most of history), people had no concept of microbes and germs. Previous cultures believed food poisonings and other diseases were caused by evil spirits, evil spells and curses. If one does not understand how systems work, then one becomes superstitious in an attempt to have control. One also becomes fearful because "good luck charms" don't control circumstances. These fears lead people to destructive behavior. It is so important to have a correct sense of cause and effect: to know how systems work.

Many cultures have their dietary "laws" rooted in ancient times when there was no refrigeration or other ways of preserving food. Later, those who survived by eating a certain way became convinced that what kept them healthy now kept them holy as well. Others followed their example.

Most Hindus, for example, practice some form of vegetarianism as a part of their religion. A Hindu friend explained to me that if a person eats a vegetable dish that was a little old, they would not get nearly as ill as if they had eaten a meat dish that was a little old. Where there is little or no food preservation, such a distinction keeps people very much alive.

From an *extension* of life standpoint, it's wise to eat a wide variety of foods. From a *quality* of life standpoint, it's also wise to eat a wide variety of foods. Why take a chance on missing something you like or need? We can learn a lot from other cultures and their habits.

In most countries, eating is an event in and of itself. The preparation and care that goes into each meal is extraordinary. Cooks consider themselves experts and are thrilled to have appreciative subjects sample their art form. In many towns, people shop every day for the ingredients that go into their meals. In their homes are the teeniest refrigerators you have ever seen – and these are for families of five. I had a bigger one in my dorm room.

Here in the U.S., many of us have at least one full- sized refrigerator in the kitchen and another freezer or refrigerator in the garage. We can feed the 8th Army and yet we hear the familiar whine over and over: "There's nothing good to eat in the house."

We eat on the run constantly, and even in restaurants, we ask for the check when the entrée arrives. In Europe, if you don't spend at least one hour talking after the meal, the proprietor will ask you if something was wrong or if someone offended you in some way. They are horrified to think that we eat *standing up* and even over the kitchen sink. Barbaric!

When our recent ancestors came to America, they thought the streets would be paved with gold. Many of them left the "old country" because of famine. So what did they do, as soon as they could, when they got here? They wanted to eat like royalty. They made corned beef sandwiches that were two inches thick and were so full you had to have *two* pieces of bread to hold it all in. Back home, a "sandwich" was a single piece of bread with a single piece of shaved meat (for the lucky), along with some other spread. Now, in the US, we call them tea sandwiches and eat them as appetizers before we get to the *real* meal. This attitude can cause us to eat far more than we need.

The Lottery, Part I

In terms of human history, we have hit the food lottery. No one in the history of the world has such an abundance of the "stuff of life" as we do right now. Not even Napoleon had the choices that we have today. No wonder you are overwhelmed.

Think about your great-great-great grandmother and her rough clothes and worn hands. Her Everest was clear. It was to keep herself and her children healthy enough to live long enough so *you could be here today*. Do you think she could envision, as she spent her time by her cooking pot at a dirt hearth, what your life would be like right now? Could she even conceive of the richness of your life: of even being able to *read* the directions on a *package* of food? What are you going to do today that would make her proud?

A lot of people use "I/He/She grew up in The Depression," as an excuse for personality quirks. This was a horrible time in our history with widespread starvation and suffering. But it is also the basis for superstitious behavior like the inability to throw away a glass jar or paper bag. It excuses people for retaining these non-serving habits.

My recent ancestors lived so far back in the country, the depression didn't affect their eating habits. When I asked Grandma what her life was like back then, she replied, "Nothing much happens around here." Their lives were simple and hard, but they lived by the seasons without many economic or political concerns.

Now is a good time for you to ask yourself, "What will I do if the money runs out?" I don't mean a complete economic collapse. There are systems in place to make sure that is unlikely. But what will happen if your company's customers go elsewhere? What other resources do you have in your lemonade stand to keep you from getting some strange personality quirks of your own?

Conventional Wisdom

A lot of what we believe about how the world works comes to us in the form of sayings and adages. Much of it is true – but a lot of it is just plain superstition. When you were five and making an ugly face, if your mom had said, "That face is making you look ugly and people are going to judge you by it" – would it still have had the same effect as, "Your face will freeze like that?" Probably not.

We call those things "old wives' tales" because we take them with a grain of salt. At least the "old wives" were really trying to change behavior to help us. A lot of our "wisdom" now comes from the media. The purpose of the media is to inform, but also to change our behavior. And unfortunately, this change in behavior is usually not for our specific benefit. The beneficiary of that change is the advertiser who delivered you the message. These messages try to convince us that we have defects that their products can cure. For example, "cellulite cures." There are creams that are guaranteed to make cellulite disappear. My feeling is that if cellulite – this vital part of a woman's anatomy – were to disappear, then so would the human race. Anti-bacterial soap is another example. Soap, by its very definition kills bacteria *already*, but advertisers can scare people into thinking their ingredients are better. Manipulating people's fears is a very old profession. There are thousands of these examples all throughout history.

According to food industry researchers, companies compete for consumer dollars by encouraging people to eat when they aren't hungry and keep eating after they are full. Food industry trade groups counter that they sell a wide variety of foods, including regular, low-calorie, reduced-fat, and sugar-free food options. They also contend that they spend more time and money advertising the low- and reduced-calorie foods than other items. Despite the advertising efforts, you need to choose *for yourself* what foods you need, and where you want to get them. Don't let them choose for you. You need to put *yourself* in an environment that encourages healthy eating and activity levels. No one else will do it for you.

Current Cultures

Not everybody looks at food the way you do. The way you look at yourself, your food and everything else has been colored by your experiences up until this very moment. The term for this is "bias." There is no such thing as "unbiased opinion" because everyone's opinions and beliefs are molded by their experiences. How can it be otherwise? We have biases toward food because of our experiences with food.

For example, I used to really dislike tomatoes before I realized I had never really had one. When I was growing up, I was usually served those under-ripe, gassed tomatoes that you find in fast-food places. They taste like cardboard. Then, one day on the Eastern Shore in Maryland, I was with a friend who was eating the most amazing dish I had ever seen. It was a *real* tomato, served with a little olive oil, salt and fresh ground pepper. It was a gorgeous shade of red and so juicy it didn't need any other dressing. It was delicious and changed the way I looked at tomatoes forever.

Another example is cucumbers. On a patio in Greece, overlooking the exquisitely blue Aegean Sea, I was served a dish of cucumber spears, dressed in the freshest olive oil, the most fragrant vinegar, salt and fresh ground pepper. To this day, I can't look at a cucumber without smelling that air and feeling that breeze.

And spinach! Everyone hates spinach. But I had it baked in an incredible breakfast casserole in a café at the base of Aspen Mountain. I could see the snow swirling around the mountain against the steel-gray sky while I sat, warm and dry on a soft banquet, waiting for the sun to come out. Do you see why I love food?

There is only one place to get such a tomato, cucumber or spinach: your local farmers market. I have never seen great tomatoes, cucumbers or spinach anywhere else. My local grocery has a great selection of fruits and vegetables, but I will still stop at the produce stand with a trunk full of frozen food to get their tomatoes, cucumbers and spinach. I won't go in to the health benefits of good produce, but it benefits every organ in your body. You can stop by your produce stand – they don't advertise – and pick up some ingredients for some great memories of your own.

The French

A lot of us look to the French with envy. How can they eat all that rich food and still stay slim? It's called the French Paradox and it's easy to understand. French cuisine is the culmination of a thousand years of daily practice, and I think they've got it down. Their choice and use of ingredients is what makes their cuisine extraordinary.

There are other factors at work, but the fat content is what most people focus on first. The French use a large number of fat *emulsifiers* in their dishes and they work in wonderful ways.

Mustards are emulsifiers. Have you ever made salad dressing from oil and vinegar? The oil floats to the top. No matter how hard you shake it, in the millisecond it takes to pour it on, the dressing separates and all you get is a plateful of oil. Now, add a teeny bit of mustard – it doesn't matter if it's dry or "prepared." The vinegar and oil mix almost immediately. Adding the bit of mustard is all it takes to emulsify the fat in the oil. Now, who has a culture of "mustard worship?" It's the folks with the Grey Poupon. There are shops in Europe totally devoted to mustards that have been in business for hundreds of years. They also invented the nubby shower massagers – pure genius!

Wine also emulsifies fat. Have you ever sautéed fish, chicken or beef and then made a sauce out of the bits left in the pan? The first step to making the sauce is to add a little wine in a process called deglazing. This mixture is then seasoned and a tablespoon of butter is swirled in to enrich the flavor and add a sheen to it. The sauce is poured over the main dish and the results are delicious.

I can hear the anti-fat freaks now, "Oh my god! Fat and butter! Do thirty sit-ups, now!!" I have a friend whose grandmother came from France and was horrified at the thought of not having wine with her evening meal. She believed that if you didn't have wine with a meal, the food would congeal in the stomach and cause all sorts of gastrointestinal problems. Wine breaks down fat and suspends it into an emulsion: you can see this for yourself when you deglaze a cooking pan. When fat is suspended into an emulsion, it has more surface area on which dietary enzymes can do their magic of digestion. The body just puts out what it doesn't need with the rest of the garbage.

The heat from the sauté pan evaporates the alcohol, so you don't have to worry about being impaired from the Sauce Bordelaise. In every good French cookbook, directions for sauces are in the very first section. It makes me crazy when I hear people tell others to eat their food without sauces. Why bother? I know I don't.

Other factors in the French Paradox are the small portion sizes we discussed earlier and the fact that gasoline is $6 a gallon. The French have trained themselves so they are not nearly so dependent on cars as we are. In fact, it is much easier to get around Paris by walking than it is to drive a car.

One major factor that almost *never* gets mentioned is that French citizens like to be educated and experienced in many different areas. In fact, instead of feeling over the hill at thirty, a French woman feels she hasn't even hit her stride until she is in her forties. And French men are very appreciative of a woman who knows how to live well. I think if the prize you are after is a good life, you don't need to worry about your weight.

So there you have it. If you are extremely satisfied with your life and your food, eat less and walk more – you won't put on extra pounds. Isn't that simple? I do it and you can, too!

East Asia

While I haven't had the pleasure of visiting East Asia (yet), I have a great respect for the cultures and foods that I have experienced through my East Asian friends. East Asian meals are almost exclusively composed of a wide variety of vegetables and grains.

The wok was invented in this region. It is ingenious for conserving energy. Instead of a flat pan that radiates heat upward, the sloping sides radiate heat back into the food to cook it more quickly. Quick cooking combined with the small size of the ingredients create fast and healthful meals. Get any wok cookbook and you can give new meaning to the phrase "fast food." You will truly appreciate your large plastic cutting board and your big chef's knife when you can whip out a delicious meal that meets your nutritional needs in less time than it takes to go pick something up at the local fast-food joint.

A good Japanese meal typically includes eight colors. Serving sizes are very small, but delicious. Traditionally, the Japanese try to eat thirty different foods per day. Now that is variety!

A typical home meal in China is almost completely without fat. It consists of a large portion of rice topped with steamed or stir-fried vegetables, tofu and/or fruit. Tofu is made from soybeans and comes in different consistencies. It takes on the flavors of the food it is cooked with and is an excellent source of protein. Meat, fish and other animal products are a rare luxury in some regions. The health benefits from different soy products are well documented. I like to take nutritional cues from them because, as a population, they have fewer debilitating diseases than Americans do.

For most of the world, food is a *tool* for nourishment and pleasure. You can widen your horizons on many levels by looking into cookbooks featuring other cultural cuisines. Head for the cookbook aisle in the library and be transported to faraway places, as well as receiving benefits from a wide variety of foods.

International Ways With Leftovers

Other cultures don't call them leftovers or plan-overs or some other contrived name. The French call them "re-heated" foods. I call them delicious. If you are not a member of the "Clean-Plater Club," you need to be an expert at using up the foods you have without eating them all at once.

It is no coincidence that the only guy I ever met who didn't eat leftovers also is the only guy I ever met who had his stomach stapled. I am an expert with leftovers – they don't have to be eaten in the same form as the night before. You just need to look at different cultures around the world. What we might consider a delicacy could be considered a routine meal in another country.

For example, if you have a big piece of meat to cook, but realize it's way more than you need, you can split it up in a number of ways. Try dividing it between a roast and cubed meat for shish kabobs on another day. When part of the roast is cooking, cut up the rest into small chunks and drop it in some marinade. The next day, skewer the meat along with a big selection of vegetables and cook under a broiler. Serve it over long grain and wild rice and you have a dinner fit for the best of company. Or try cutting the meat into strips and make fajitas later in the week.

As simple as it is, it does take a little planning, so here are some ideas to get you started. The recipes are in <u>Chapter 13</u>.

American-style: Use leftover meat or poultry for a grilled sandwich, sandwich salad or a main dish salad. Leftover barbequed chicken is great in a chicken-salad sandwich recipe and thinly sliced leftover steak is a treat in a green salad with either Parmesan or soy-ginger dressing.

Mexican-style: Wrap leftovers in a tortilla with condiments. Any kind of sautéed meat, chicken or vegetable is great served with rice and beans. Sometimes I just use leftover black beans and rice by itself. I put these out with salsa, chopped tomato, chopped lettuce, green onion, shredded cheese and sliced avocado or guacamole. Everyone takes flour tortillas and rolls their own creation.

English-style: Bake last night's dinner in a pastry-lined pie plate or make Shepard's Pie. You can get frozen piecrust shells at the grocer and use them instead of homemade paté brisee (pie crust dough). Let the piecrust thaw on the counter while you make a filling of sauce and whatever else you have on hand. Bake for 25 minutes and you're done. If you don't want to mess with a piecrust, put the filling in a casserole and spoon leftover mashed potatoes or Bisquick biscuits on top before baking.

Korean and Japanese-style: Roll some sushi. Sushi is simply different kinds of ingredients (cooked or raw) rolled up with sushi rice in dried seaweed sheets. Sushi rice is very sticky, short-grained rice mixed with a little rice vinegar and sesame oil that holds the sushi roll together. You can use avocado, asparagus, green beans, mushrooms, cucumber, carrot, real or artificial crabmeat, caviar, cooked spinach, sliced scrambled egg, cooked shrimp, tofu – almost anything. This is an ancient art and it's best to have someone teach you in person instead of trying to learn it from a cookbook. But when you get the hang of it, people will be clamoring for your leftovers – I promise.

French-style: Heat leftovers in cream sauce and serve over a fancy type of toast or crepes – or try making omelets. You can keep commercial puff pastry shells and / or homemade crepes in the freezer. Crepes are ingenious because they are very thin batter pancakes cooked either on the *inside or outside* of the pan. I make them every so often and keep a stack ready to wrap around ham and asparagus. Add a little Swiss cheese and it looks like you worked for hours.

Far Eastern-style: Make fried rice. I usually make a double batch of rice and make fried rice later in the week to use up all my leftovers. I stir-fry different raw vegetables, add the rice, some sauce and bits of leftover beef, pork or chicken and a few of those tiny frozen shrimp (I don't know what else to do with them). My family really thinks this is special and I remember my daughter saying to her dad, "Look what we get!" as if the stir-fry I had put together was a holiday meal.

Middle East-style: Skewer some kabobs. You can make a million varieties of kabobs with whatever fruits, vegetables and meats that you have on hand. Soak some bamboo skewers in water and make up whatever combination suits your fancy.

American South–style: Sauté some vegetables (carrots, celery and onion) with some herbs. Add a can of black-eyed peas and some leftover chopped ham. Serve over rice with tomato, green onion and shredded cheese. This dish is called Hoppin' John, and with a side of corn bread, it is heavenly.

American North-style: Brown some ground meat in a large pan. Add a couple of cans of tomato sauce and whatever else you have. I use mushrooms, zucchini and leftover corn. Let it simmer for about twenty minutes, then mix in some cooked macaroni and top with shredded cheese. My friends in the frozen north call this "hot dish" and it is very comforting on a lousy day.

There are thousands of different soup and stew recipes available. Keep a selection of herbs and spices to best complement the taste of your foods and you can't go wrong. If you still don't think you can transform any old leftover into a great meal, maybe this little story will convince you.

I keep something called "dried chipped beef" on hand, which is the polar opposite of anything "gourmet." My sister, the chef, was complaining that her family wasn't appreciating her. To commiserate, I said that I make only "chipped beef on toast" when I felt unappreciated. She thought it was a great idea and said as we hung up, "That'll fix them. They'll only get chipped beef tonight!" Well, of course, she had to put a little tarragon and other good ingredients in it. She was flabbergasted when her family raved about the dried chipped beef she expected them to complain about – and now they request it often. It doesn't matter what you start with, only that if you prepare your food carefully and serve it lovingly, you will get great results. Having a thousand ways to use up leftovers means that you are *always* eating well.

Local Sub-Cultures

It's easy to see that other cultures around the world are different from our own. But did you ever stop to think that there might be other cultures in your own backyard? These are groups of people, your neighbors, with similar hobbies and lifestyles. You might find it wise to have one or two different groups of people to "hang out" with. They could have ways of doing things that might be of benefit to you.

Skinny people, for instance. If someone asks you to go for a walk, it might benefit you to go once or twice instead of looking shocked (as has happened to me). Who knows? If you've been out of it, you might pick up the walking habit again. Or you could do the asking.

Sometimes it just doesn't work out. I couldn't hack it when I tried to hang out with a group of people who eschewed red meat and alcohol and ran marathons for fun. I really liked them a lot and they liked me, too, but I had to find another group of friends. I just couldn't keep up. There are all kinds of clubs and groups you can join or start yourself so you can add more of what *you* need to your life.

For example, I love scuba diving. Going diving is a workout in itself, but nobody notices because it's so much fun. After a couple of months of lugging heavy equipment around (everyone has to carry their own) and proper breathing, there's no way a person can stay out of shape. Toning up is automatic because weight training and cardio are built right into the fun. The folks in my scuba diving clubs are in great shape. It's hard to believe, but we never lack for volunteers for the beachwear fashion show.

There must be dozens of groups you'd like to join around your town. Do not let your fears of being out of shape or looking foolish deter you. I can hear you saying now, "I was always picked last in gym class!" Well, I was, too. As a matter of fact, I don't know anyone who was *ever* picked first. Are you going to let the opinion of someone you didn't know well then and don't know *at all* anymore stop you from doing what you want for fun?

If you are out of shape now, that is *exactly* what you are doing. You are letting others have control over you that they do not deserve. STOP IT!!

DO NOT let that attitude stop you from having better relationships, a better body and a longer life that you enjoy. This is exactly what you are giving up if you put your life on hold until you lose five pounds!! It's not worth it.

Widen your radar screen and go find groups that will make you think and feel, "We are doing something great!" If your current culture isn't encouraging you to eat well and stay active – go find another group that will.

Chapter 10

Eating Right by Sight:
The "Italian Flag" Diet

Is money important to you? Of course it is. Quick! The last three checks you wrote: Who were they to and how much were they for? Of course, you don't remember. You can't remember what you had for dinner a week ago Thursday, either. So why do you think you can keep track of everything you eat? I am *not* suggesting writing it down, but just as those who don't overspend have an idea about how much they can afford, those who are not overweight have an idea about what and how much they are eating.

That's why it's so important to think out what it is that you are going to eat when you get hungry. You *are* going to get hungry and, if you are lucky, it's going to happen several times a day. I get hungry about five times a day. And then I eat.

Take a good hard look at what is in your refrigerator and freezer right now. I know I am in trouble when all I see is coffee, nuts, ice blocks and bait. Then I know I need to sit down for an hour and figure out what I want to eat, as well as what I want to feed my family and friends. If I don't do that planning, it's back to fast-food alley – and we all know where that leads!

I used to think planning meals was like financial planning: you drag out all of your records, pore over the information, make a plan, and stick to it. You can't *do* that in the real world. In a regular household, you only deal with money five to ten times a day. You deal with 30 to 40 food choices every day just for yourself. That doesn't include the choices involved in managing a family, too. You could never get up from the table if you tried to follow that example.

But, to make your food choices work for you and not against you, you need to make your choices *ahead of time*.

In Chapter 6, I discussed the importance of making some arbitrary choices. In Chapter 8, I explained how food choices affect the quality of your life. Now we are going to start to put it all together.

The thought of "planning menus in advance" conjures up images of a person sitting down at a table with a stack of cookbooks, trying to put together a weekly feast. Who has time for that? A professional chef maybe, but not anyone I know. To me, planning menus means having a second list next to the grocery list of the dishes I can make because I've got all the ingredients on hand.

Most people have rotating periods of frenzy and relative calm in their lives. Just remember that emergencies and uncontrollable situations *will* happen. Simple planning will make what you *want* to eat available.

Planning vs. Scheduling, Part II

People often confuse the two concepts of planning and scheduling. You plan a vacation, but schedule a haircut. Most people plan to exercise, but they don't schedule it. Many nutritionists lecture about meal planning – but so many of us confuse it with meal scheduling.

My meal planning is knowing what I can make for dinner during the upcoming week and what ingredients I need. Before grocery shopping once a week, I make a list of five dinners. I then buy the necessary ingredients and pick one meal when I need to put dinner on the table. I don't throw those lists away. I reuse them all the time because it's hard enough to put together *one* meal, much less a healthy new one every day that the whole family enjoys. The same goes for breakfast, lunch and snacks, too.

I *don't* say to myself: "Well, I'll put the chicken in the oven on Sunday at 6 p.m., the meatloaf can be made on Monday, etc..." My approach is, "I c an fix spaghetti, chicken Caesar salad, or…" Then it's easy to look at the list so I can eat what *I* want to eat.

When meals are pre-planned and ready to go, it's sort of like looking in the freezer for a frozen meal. But you'll like these meals better – and they'll likely be better for you than something you poked holes in and put in the microwave. You can schedule something besides frozen dinners and rely on your freezer stash only when it's *really* necessary. And, because meal times don't drag me down, I find time for other things that I want to do – like playing with the kids.

Planning and scheduling are about advance preparation. Not only do you have a list of what you need, but you must have some idea of what you are actually going to do with the ingredients when you get home. You plan what to buy and then schedule the actual work. You have to do both or you are wasting the time and effort you put into one or the other.

So, what do you put on the grocery list? I start by looking at what I already have on hand. This can be tricky because, very often, the foods we really like get eaten and what is left "on-hand" is stuff we don't like. It's easy to fall into that trap. You had a coupon for one of the thousands of new products that come out every year and it was so awful it never left the cupboard after the first taste.

It's important to periodically toss out the food that will likely never get eaten. The reason is this: every time you open the refrigerator or pantry door, there *it* is, staring you in the face. You're looking at food you don't like, and the next thing you know, *you are hating food again.* Get rid of it!

People try to get around throwing out these bad items by giving them to Boy Scout food drives or try to make the foods into a dish for a potluck supper. But you're not doing anyone any favors. Poor people have taste buds, too, and you don't really want your friends to think you cook like *that*, do you? Now, after you have cleared out everything you *aren't* going to eat, decide on what you *are* going to eat.

As I previously mentioned, every person lives on about ten foods. People eat the same thing over and over. Look at your own grocery list – do you find yourself buying the same foods every time you are at the store? If these foods are not helping you to be the best you can be, maybe it's time for a change. Add foods that will help you reach your goals – foods that are holding you back will drop away.

You've already looked at your vitamin needs and compared it to the foods you eat all the time. What is missing? And how do you fill it in? Read on.

Why Didn't I Think of This Before?

This is it – the cornerstone of eating right. You are going to kick yourself for not doing this sooner. ***You Need to Eat in Technicolor!!*** So many people eat sepia-toned meals: meat, potatoes and gravy, chicken and biscuits, steak and baked, etc. Where are the brilliant reds, vibrant greens and bright oranges in their lives?

Everyone needs to *add* to food choices, not take them away. Most people do the opposite. You hear the refrain every time people get together: "I can't eat this, I can't eat that." With the exception of the seriously allergic, that approach to "dieting," and life, is plain stupid.

So many people out there eat brown and white meals. Meat and potatoes are brown and white. Burgers and fries, hot dogs and chips, chicken and rice – there isn't a good color among them. Instead, look for the *Italian Flag* on your plate while you fix your food. Do you see red, white and green? This concept is so simple, but if you don't see all three colors, you need to *add* whatever is missing. In Chapter 8, I said I was convinced that withholding foods would backfire: this is how I add them.

Mother Nature color-coded her food offerings to us. For the non-chemists out there – every chemical has a certain array of colors that identify it. Generally, because vitamins are chemicals, it naturally follows that they can be identified by the colors they impart to food.

Red (or orange or yellow) foods include tomatoes, yams, strawberries, carrots, and corn. These foods are rich in vitamins A and C and are vital for good eyesight, healthy skin and joints, and maintain the linings of organs, such as lungs. How can you breath with your whole lung if the lining is tattered?

Green foods, of course, include leafy vegetables, beans, broccoli and cabbage. These are rich in minerals. If a tree is yellowing (always a bad thing: the leaves are dying), it needs some mineral to make it green again. By eating green foods, you are picking up minerals your body needs for all of those chemical reactions we discussed in Chapter 4.

The B vitamins are found in white foods. Milk, grains, eggs and yeasts in breads all contain significant amounts that help with nerve reactions and brain function.

These white foods also have proteins and carbohydrates (starches), and include pastas, potatoes, bread, nuts, eggs and rice. Other foods, including meat, fish, poultry and tofu contain *complete* proteins. If a grain, such as rice, is combined with a legume, such as beans, the combination provides the body with the amino acids that create a complete protein. These complete proteins are the building blocks of our muscles, skin, hair, and nails. Many cultures use the beans and rice combination as their main source of protein. That's why kids still grow when they live on peanut butter and jelly sandwiches.

This is also an example of why I'm not a proponent of a limited carbohydrate diet. All of these foods do so much good for the body – with few carbs, the brain and body don't receive what they need to function.

Carb Cutters are Crazy

Remember the food chain? Can you recall how all food begins in plants as light energy from the sun? This is how it works. The green chemical in plant leaves is called chlorophyll. When sunlight shines on the chlorophyll, its energy is stored within the plant like a teeny, tiny battery. When carbon dioxide (the stuff you and I breath out) enters the leaves, it combines with the energy to make a simple sugar. This sugar is then moved through the plant to form its stems, roots, fruits and seeds, forging another link in the food chain.

Now I ask you, how can you completely cut out sugar from your diet if every food in the galaxy starts out as a sugar? Well, you can't. You can only pick and choose what it is you need from your food and what else you want to go along with it.

So, as often as possible, *I eat red, white and green*. It is so easy. Look at your plate. If you see only brown and white, cut up a tomato and add some lettuce. If it's only white and red, open a can of green beans. If it's just red and green, grab a bread stick.

Ideally, you should eat as many colors as possible. It's the easiest way to "eat a balanced diet." This may be an oversimplification, but like anything else, eating differently takes practice. If you've been sleepwalking through your meals, you need to start simple. Later, take some time to look around and really think about what you want to live on. Expanding your horizons and incorporating many different foods in your diet won't just help your health. It will give you more energy. It will affect your appearance. It will make you more interesting. Don't believe me? As a make-up artist, I noticed that people with the best skin enjoyed their vegetables. And good skin is a major indicator of good health. It's also a lot more interesting to talk to someone about a great meal than to hear someone say, "I can't eat this, I can't eat that."

Eating well will give you energy, make you more attractive and contribute to better health. And if you have your health, you have everything.

My Grocery List

Here I'm going to show you some of the items that appear most often on my grocery list. The 10 things I live on include:

1. Rice, lots of different rice – yellow, black beans and rice, sushi rice, brown rice, wild rice
2. Pasta
3. Tortilla wraps
4. Breakfast cereal, usually something with an oat
5. Fresh fruits and vegetables
6. Fruit and vegetable juices
7. Cheeses
8. Eggs
9. Bread
10. Canned tuna – in oil

If I look in my pantry, refrigerator and freezer right now, I have eight different kinds of rice, six kinds of pasta, three types of tortillas, four breakfast cereals (two with oats), 15 kinds of fresh fruits and vegetables and even more types that are canned, eight kinds of cheese, a dozen eggs, six cans of tuna (in oil) and seven types of bread. I also have different kinds of beef, chicken, pork and shellfish that are canned, frozen and fresh. It sounds like a lot, but I *do* have a family to feed.

Just about everything I cook or eat has at least one of these ingredients in it. I use them to make soups and stews, sandwiches, stir-fries, salads, wraps and one-dish meals. I may shop for specific items for special meals, but I can't and don't do that every day.

Chapter 12, <u>The Skinny Girl Cooks</u>, will provide you with ideas for meals and help you set up your kitchen. You really can fix an excellent meal for yourself and your family for less money and in less time than it takes to go through the drive through. A few weeks ago, I spent $15 at a fast food restaurant – and the fries were lousy. What a waste! I could have gotten a lot more for my $15 if I had thought about it earlier.

There are recipes for foods at every stage of the freshness curve. Believe it or not, I don't *like* to throw food away, so I have a few recipes that will stretch the useful life of some foods.

At the grocery store, all the good red, white and green foods are on the outside walls. Most people go into the store, turn right and then start weaving through the aisles – up one and down the other – through the processed food. If I do that, my grocery budget is shot before I get to the fruits and vegetables because I have to pass the frozen pizza first. It's so much better for me to make the *outside circle* first. I pass the dairy, meat, bakery and produce counters first and pick up what I need. If I'm on a tight budget, I then figure out how much I have left to spend and *only then* begin to weave through the aisles. Another bonus is that I end up at the checkouts near my car.

The tip to remember is to have your kitchen set up so making a delicious meal can become the *easiest and cheapest* thing for you to do. You can't eat good food unless you have it within arms reach.

For years, I have wanted to tell the manager of my local market to put up a sign that says in huge letters: "They Can't Eat Vegetables If You Don't Buy Them!" They also need to have little tear-off pads of recipes so customers can put vegetable dishes together with as little fuss as a microwave dinner or a Lunchables.

Convenience stores, too, should be making *dinner* convenient. Based on the ads hanging inside the store, *everyone* is looking to buy eight different kinds of cigarettes and a six-pack of domestic beer. They should be competing with the fast food places by offering something people can eat every day, without regret, for the rest of their lives.

Of course, that will only happen in my personal utopia. But, we can still make finding fruits and vegetables, and creating dishes around them, part of our daily lives. If you don't know how to make those fruits and vegetables tasty, spend some time in the produce department at your local grocery. Find the foreign people who work there. Ask them how they prepare their vegetables. If the accent's not too thick, you can get some fantastic ideas.

One July, I was trying to have a Cinderella party for my daughter. There are *no* pumpkins around here in July. Desperately, I asked the produce man at my local market if there was anything he could direct me to. He said, "I have pumpkin from my country in the back. It's called calabeeza." I was so relieved that I didn't even ask him which country he was from *or* realize he had sold me his own dinner. After a bunch of 4-year-olds tried to turn the pumpkin into Cinderella's golden carriage, we cooked it and ate it. And it was delicious.

Once I took my 10-year-old neighbor on a field trip to the local produce market. Her mom does not cook and she wanted to learn about food. We went through every single fruit and vegetable in the whole place, talking about what it was, what it would do for the body and how to serve it. Today, I see her home on college breaks, picking breakfast off her family's fruit trees for her friends.

I also let kids buy anything they want in the produce department or at the farmer's market. Most of us never get the chance to let our kids pick out anything they want in a store, but it's easy at a produce stand. And you know it will be good for them. They couldn't carry more than $10 worth of fruits and vegetables if they tried. Then you can all go home and cook together. Kids are much more inclined to eat fruits and vegetables if they have picked them out and helped cook them.

I love my local produce stand. Everyone that works there *knows* food. They have the freshest produce around because it usually just came out of the ground that very morning. If you don't have a produce stand or weekly greenmarket nearby, find one or you'll be missing out.

They usually have the best prices, too. They don't advertise except on hand-lettered signs. Most of us have been trained not to accept a food that doesn't come hermetically sealed in a perfectly manufactured package or already cooked in a wrapper or on a plate. But, if you've never picked a pole bean and eaten it right there in the garden on a sunny day – you haven't lived.

When and What to Eat

I usually eat about five times a day. That's about every three hours, if I get my way. I eat breakfast within an hour of waking *every single day*, no exceptions. I usually have something with an oat in it, such as oatmeal, or an oat cereal. If I have some orange juice and some melon – there's the red, white and green that I look for – but any combination is just as good.

My fear is getting in an accident on the way to work and going hungry until after the tow truck leaves. Luckily this has never happened – probably because I'm not fuzzyheaded from not eating.

Sometimes I have a snack between breakfast and lunch, but often it's just a juice drink. Then I eat lunch, followed by another snack in the afternoon and dinner.

Don't get snacks and "snack foods" confused. What I eat for snacks, most people would call appetizers. I like my snacks to be red, white and green, too. I like to have grapes and apple wedges, cheese and juice. And I do love chips and salsa.

What is the magic of this "secret, revolutionary" diet plan? By adding red and green to your plate, the meat and potato portion is cut in half and the fruit and veggie portion is increased by an infinite factor. You begin to eat less of the foods that could cause heart disease and weight gain and more of the foods that have the necessary nutrients to keep you in top shape – *and you haven't given up a thing*!

The point is that I give myself a steady supply of high-quality fuel throughout the day. Most people don't. They skip breakfast because they think that if they eat breakfast they will feel hungry later. (I think that's the point. If you feel hungry, you are *using* energy rather than *storing* it.) These people leave the house ravenous and before two hours are up, they are looking for the nearest doughnut drive through or something from the vending machine. Do they go for the good stuff? No. They go for the densest, most calorie-laden item available because their bodies are sending the signal that they are starving. Then it's all downhill from there.

This is why candy bars and other junk foods are always by the check out counter. Merchandisers know most people haven't thought about what they are going to eat. When they feel hunger, that hand will reach out and put the candy bar on the counter. It has to. Your body *has* to go on autopilot to survive and it's out of your conscious control. I have heard people talk about binging and stuffing themselves until they are comatose and it's *always* on a white food. It's never pineapple.

I don't know what binging means. I don't have or need willpower to resist junk foods, but I don't overeat because I just don't have to.

That's why you should eat before you leave the house. Don't eat in the car. And try not to eat from the limited selection from the vending machine. If you eat first thing in the morning, you won't be hungry for a huge jelly doughnut at 10 a.m. When the pastry platter is in the break room, *have some.* You can. Have all you want. But, if you stop when you're full, you'll probably only have eaten half or less of a pastry. *Leave the rest on the platter or throw it away.* If you indulge every day, the pastry will become one of your staple foods. It isn't providing you any nutritional benefit and you will have to adjust your eating habits accordingly or you could balloon up in a few years.

So there you have it – an easy way to ensure good nutrition. Look at your vitamins, check what's missing and add as many colors to your plate as you possibly can. How could it be simpler? And how can you go wrong?

To add more foods, try to fill in some of the blanks. If you can't, head to the produce stand!

Green foods I like are:

1.

2.

3.

Red foods I like are:

1.

2.

3.

Grains I like are: _____

Oats
Wheat
Rye
Corn
Rice

I eat them in: _____

I eat _____ for breakfast on most days.

I would like to eat:

1.

2.

3.

Chapter 11

My Favorite Fats

Oh boy, what a sore subject this is. You would think that fat was a four-letter curse word by the way people talk about it and avoid it like the plague. But the misinformation and misapplied knowledge of fat has done the worst damage to countless metabolisms.

Too much of the wrong fat can kill you. Too little of the right fat can kill you, too. Where do you draw the line?

Believe it or not, it was not so long ago that people didn't get *enough* fat in their diets. There was even a *fat crisis* in the U.S. in the 1920s and 1930s. The government began an information campaign to encourage people to eat more fat to stay healthy. Cooks devised recipes to wring every calorie possible from meat products. They held competitions for the best lard sculpture. Really, some still practice this art form today.

But, as you saw in <u>Chapter 9</u>, for most of us, our culture is entirely different than it was back then. At the start of the 1900s, nearly half of our population was in the business of producing food. Now, just <u>1</u> percent of our population feeds the entire country and a good deal of the rest of the world, too. There is *no reason* why people should be going hungry anywhere anymore.

Having enough to eat every day is a new thing by world standards. History has programmed our bodies to think, "Famine! Famine! I have to conserve my energy until my next meal." And that is exactly what it does. People who skip breakfast often enough don't get hungry in the morning because their metabolisms have slowed to help them cope with starvation.

When the body goes into the famine mode, it gets very stingy about giving up its energy stores and slows down metabolic processes. Fuel, circulating in the blood from the last meal, is used up within four to six hours. The body then begins to enter its starvation mode by using fuel it has stored in the liver. Six to twelve hours after its last meal, when *that* fuel is exhausted, the body begins to rapidly make fuel from *muscle protein* – not fat.

As we mentioned previously, over-eating is a way of life for many people. (They're in the Clean-Plater Club.) But after these individuals store up those calories, they try to deal with the extra weight by not eating. Wrong, wrong, wrong!! The body will not even *begin* to tap fat stores until it has been starving for *two weeks*. By that time a huge amount of muscle mass, which best metabolizes energy, has been permanently lost.

This is why diets don't work. The very thing you need to burn fat – your muscles – are used up first to keep your body going. When you start eating again, there is less muscle to metabolize the energy from your food and your body wisely stores the excess as fat for your next bout of starvation. You can't lose weight *and have a life* by not eating. It won't work, so don't try it. If it was easy and possible, people would lose weight and that would be the end of it.

My 119-pound body has no concern for its next meal. I love my food and I give my body the best I can in terms of nutrition and taste. My body knows I would never starve it and my metabolism never slows. It has to stay high for me to *live* my life. I know I'm giving it what it needs. I rarely have to tap the stored fuel and my muscles stay in great shape so I can eat as much as I want *and* enjoy it, too.

One thing my body really needs is the right kind of fat. Maybe we should just call it oil. Everyone knows what happens to cars when they have no oil: engines freeze up and die. When you take your car to a mechanic, he goes through the list of oils – the good quality, and the not-so-good quality. You get better performance from the good quality oils. The oils *you* consume are no different. If your weight isn't where you want it to be, among other things, you should *change your oil*.

You *need* fat in your diet to allow the absorption of certain vitamins and minerals into the blood stream to nourish the cells in your body. These vitamins and minerals bind with cell pollution to slow the aging process, prevent the plaque that can form in the arteries and veins and reduce the risks of heart disease, stroke, cancer and other life-shortening disasters. Without the proper oil, these so-called "fat soluble" vitamins can't get to where they need to be to benefit you. Myelin, the "insulation" on your nerve cells is made of a type of fat as well.

At one time, I studied different kinds of fat and discovered that some were indeed vital and others vile. Though I'm not a chemist, as an interested consumer, I have found that the Center for Science on the Public Interest (www.cspinet.org) has a lot of good information on different fats necessary for proper nutrition. Please remember that writers are never neutral about nutrition information. People have unavoidable biases for or against different foods, ranging from their experiences in childhood to who is paying for their current research. It's wise to get all the information you can (within reason) to help you make the food decisions that are best for you. Keep in mind that common words can get mixed up with the meanings of scientific terms like "saturation," "salts" and "acid." I've given you my criteria for picking good foods, but I am sure you can come up with other ideas of your own.

Fat Is Where the Flavor Is

It seems that all the taste of food is bound up in its fats. If you remove the fat from a dish, the flavor evaporates. For this reason, I don't eat "low fat" anything. It has no taste for me. If I pick up something low fat by mistake, I go back and get the regular thing before I waste my time and money. I have already decided how much fat I want to eat. Instead of spreading mayo on a sandwich like cake frosting, I use enough to get the taste I want. I don't eat low calorie items, either. Why bother drinking a beer if it has no taste? I'll have the water if there is only light beer to be had.

If there is too much fat in my meal, it becomes too rich for me and I can only eat a couple of bites before feeling full. You can experiment with different types of fat in your staple foods. Just because I don't care for 2 percent milk doesn't mean that *you* shouldn't drink it if you want to.

The Good, the Bad and the Ugly

A good fat is going to give you smooth skin and glossy hair. It will help you think more clearly and shorten your reaction time. A bad fat will clog your arteries and slow you down. Ugly fat is...well, everywhere. Do I have to describe it?

Oils that are liquid at room temperature are necessary, but some of those oils are more vital than others, and as with anything, overuse can cause problems. Choose wisely. For example, fish oils contain omega 3 fatty acids, one of the most important nutrients for brain development. In an experiment, baby monkeys given infant formula containing omega 3 fatty acids were more alert and stronger than baby monkeys given regular baby formula.

Omega 3 fatty acids are found in fish, nuts, flax seeds, soybeans and canola oil. Omega 3s are one of many "fat soluble" compounds that need to dissolve in oil to be carried by the blood stream. They *can't* dissolve in water and it is my belief that you do not get the benefit of these vital compounds if you eat only "water-packed fish." Also, certain fats have the ability to remove artery-clogging debris. If this debris is made of fat, it makes sense to me that a "good" fat is needed to dissolve the debris in order for it to be carried away. This concept will be familiar to you if you have ever taken a grease stain out of a shirt by "reactivating" it with another oil and then washing it out.

The fats to avoid are *solid at room temperature*. These include natural fats *and* man-made fats. Solid animal fats can clog arteries in no time. These natural fats adorn pieces of meat and sit in tubs of lard. Man-made fats such as solid margarines and shortenings have been "hydrogenated" during their production to create a solid or semi-solid form. The fat molecules receive extra hydrogen atoms during the process of *hydrogenation*. Although this may sound innocent, hydrogenation makes "trans-fatty acids" that can cause certain compounds to adhere to blood vessel linings, making them narrower and susceptible to clogging. There is solid research indicating that thousands of premature deaths from heart disease could be avoided every year if polyunsaturated fats were substituted for trans-fats.

You know I pick out foods with my circulation in mind. Sometimes I look at foods and wonder how my heart would pump that sludge through my veins. I hate the thought of a lot of fat creeping it's way around the organs in my gut like the fat in a piece of prime rib. I can't stand the thought of my poor heart and liver trying to do their vital jobs for me in that kind of environment.

With that thought in mind, it's really *easy* to leave that big hunk of solid fat (no matter what the disguise) on the plate and go for the vegetable soup. When you look at labels, leave the hydrogenated oils on the shelf. When you get out a fat gram counter, you can see that beneficial fats can easily be substituted for risky fats.

My Favorite Fats

The fats I use on a regular basis are olive oil, canola oil, peanut oil, sweet butter, and squeeze and spray margarine. I even make my own mayonnaise once in a while with peanut or olive oil. I also use a small amount of butter-flavored shortening for baking.

Olive oil is a staple in Mediterranean cuisines, and there are as many flavors of olive oil as there are of wine. Some are light, others are heavy and some fall in between. My family prefers the taste of light olive oils in salad dressings and on bruschetta (bread topped with garlic and vegetables). I like the fuller flavored oils for dipping.

Olives and their oils have been in use since before the advent of written language. The Greeks named their capital city of Athens after the goddess Athena, to thank her for giving them the olive for food, heat, light, medicine and beauty preparations.

Olive oil contains more than a hundred recognized compounds. Some of these are vital to good health. Unfortunately heating can destroy many of them, so it's important to look for extra-virgin olive oil. It's even better if it is "cold pressed." Virgin and pure olive oils can be processed in a number of ways that might harm the compounds. They are certainly better than other oils out there, but you might be missing the benefits of cold-pressed, extra-virgin olive oil if you never use it. Any good Italian, Greek or Spanish cookbook should offer a primer on olive oils and their use.

Cooking with some olive oils can be challenging because of their low smoke point. Extra-virgin olive oils can't be heated to a temperature as high as other oils. In other words, it can burn easily and ruin your dish. I think a lot of people try olive oil and get turned off after using it incorrectly or sampling a flavor they don't like.

On the other hand, peanut oil, an unsaturated fat, has an extremely high smoking point and is ideal for frying. When the cold food hits the hot peanut oil, a mini explosion takes place, effectively sealing the surface of the food to prevent oil from soaking in. This is the secret to a great tempura, the popular Japanese dish. If the oil is not hot enough, the oil seeps right in and makes the food greasy.

Canola oil doesn't come from canolas. It comes from seeds that have been crossbred to produce an oil with all of the benefits and few of the risks of other seed oils. It is also less expensive than peanut oil. I use it when a recipe calls for a tablespoon or two of oil.

Canola oil is an extraordinarily well-balanced source of the fatty acids, linoleic acid and linolenic acid. These two are essential for the health of the entire body because they are the building blocks of compounds that regulate the flow of every system. This includes water and electrolytes, temperature, blood flow to the brain, kidneys and through arteries, as well as blood pressure, bronchial tone (air flow in lungs), protection from stomach acid and intestinal efficiency, and male and female fertility. By having the right balance of fatty acids in your diet, you might be able to empty an entire shelf in the medicine cabinet.

Oils are great in cooking, but there is nothing like butter. I keep real butter in the fridge, and a pound in the freezer, too. My family consumes about a pound every month, which is one stick a week for the entire family. A tablespoon here and a tablespoon there add a lot of flavor and not a lot of fat grams. I love different kinds of butter, but I usually buy unsalted because I enjoy the flavor.

There are as many kinds of butter as there are cows. The grass they graze, or rather the diets of the cows, flavor the butter produced from their cream. European butters are heavenly. Denmark, France and England have been making butter for thousands of years, and you can buy it right at your gourmet market. Irish butter has a tang to it. I can't find it here in the States, but I enjoy it when I go abroad. Those "no-fat" people probably don't know that butter even has "flavors." They are missing out.

We typically use squeeze and spray margarine rather than the tub variety. These liquid fats have fewer hydrogenated oils and can't solidify, and they're easier to put on foods – no knives. The spray margarine is purely for flavor – there are zeros in all of the nutrient and fat columns on the label. I love a squirt on lightly steamed spinach.

Somehow people used to think that solid margarine was better for you than butter, but I think it can cause all kinds of nasty things to happen to your insides that are even worse than what a little butter can do. Butter is a naturally occurring saturated fat and has been in worldwide use for thousands of years. Solid margarine is a relatively *recent* culinary development.

Most solid margarines have had extra hydrogen atoms attached and become saturated trans-fats. Trans means "across." These fats have hydrogen molecules on *both* sides (instead of only one side) and are straight as boards. By stacking like cord wood, they become solid at room temperature *and* very stable. This stability allows them to prevent food spoilage and enables companies to give a "freshness guarantee." But it also causes them to wreak havoc with our systems.

The body has certain enzymes and compounds that are capable of dealing with a small amount of natural saturated fat by bonding with and metabolizing the fats. Unfortunately, our bodies have no way to deal with a man-made fat that has only recently been introduced into modern diets. These straight molecules are of similar size and weight to natural fats (Only the shape is different.), and the body attempts to use them in cell membranes. But because our enzymes, which work like keys in locks, don't recognize the shape, they have the effect of throwing a monkey wrench into the works by not metabolizing efficiently.

The big problem is that trans fats are everywhere these days. Look for the word <u>hydrogenation</u> on food labels and keep them out of your staple foods. Another type of fat to stay away from is LDL cholesterol. The first LD means "low-density." Think of it as "lethal dryer lint" that can cause big problems if it clogs up your ductwork. Other types of cholesterol are helpful and the body will make its own if it needs to.

For baking, I use butter-flavored shortening in recipes and cooking spray to grease my pans. I use liquid oils in other foods because they taste better. For example, sesame oil is like perfume to me. It has a "sweet-roasted" scent. It should be added at the end of cooking – like just before serving a stir-fry or in dishes like cold sesame noodles, a pasta dish served with a lot of accompaniments like cucumber and peanuts.

I also buy *real cheese*, not cheese food. Cheese food is not real food because it is loaded with artificial fats, as well as questionable fat substitutes. Nothing satisfies like real cheese and there should be only three or four *natural* ingredients on the label.

An indulgence for me is homemade mayonnaise. You can make it with either peanut or olive oil and there is nothing like it. Europeans make their own mayonnaise frequently – it's nothing like the pasty stuff you see in American supermarkets. Europeans are so crazy about "Pommes Frites avec Mayonnaise," (French fries with sauce) that they have French fry stands everywhere like we have hot dog stands. Real French fries are made in a process called "double-frying." The fries are cooked once until they are slightly brown, removed from the hot oil and allowed to rest for a while. Just before serving they are plunged into the hot oil for a few seconds for a final browning. They are so crispy on the outside and tender on the inside that if you ever have them, you'll never want to buy fast-food fries again.

Quick Reaction Times

Our bodies require the right kinds of fats for survival. If the myelin sheath coating your nerve cells is tattered, the messages traveling down them can short circuit. The messages don't reach the intended destination and your body can't do what you want it to do. As a person ages, the nerves can degenerate in so many ways. But, if the myelin covering is in good shape, nerve impulses can reach their destinations instantaneously and reaction time gets infinitely quicker. You can sense things faster than others and that can do everything from improving mental acuity to saving a life.

One day, my daughter was visiting a friend while I was at a meeting. When the meeting was over, I went to pick her up and went inside to chat with her mom while the kids played. We were in the playroom when her two-year-old, as only a two-year-old can do, shifted a leg on a TV stand. At 30 inches, the TV took two people to lift it into place and the stand was rather flimsy. Everyone watched in horror as the TV started to topple over on the little boy. To me, it looked like it was moving in slow motion. It's weird how the mind works in tragic situations. In less than a second I was able to evaluate what would happen if the TV fell and whether or not the little boy could get out of the way in time. Even as fast as he was, I figured that he couldn't. In the next instant I found myself pushing the boy out of the way and under the weight of the TV. I can still feel my back and leg muscles screaming as *I pushed that enormous TV back up on its stand.* The others in the room could only look on with gaping mouths. Now I know how a mom can lift a Volkswagen when her child has been run over.

I shudder to think what would have happened if I had hesitated or wasn't in good shape. If I had hesitated, that TV, in the best case, would have crashed and blown glass all over the children. The worst was that the little boy might have been killed. If I hadn't hesitated but was not in good shape, I would have certainly been injured. *But that didn't happen.* What I could do in those two seconds was enough. I'm no body builder, but I was strong enough to change the course of history for myself and six other people. No one has nightmares of seeing and hearing a horrible accident. It would have ruined our lives just to watch. But, instead, when it was over, my daughter ran up to me, hugged me tight and said "Mommy, you saved his life!"

The Right Stuff

You could be harming yourself if you've been eating the wrong fats or avoiding them altogether. Either course is wrong. You want to think clearly, have *healthy* skin inside and out, *and* all the benefits of good circulation. Vital fats are what you need. Change your oil if you need to. You have already decided how much fat is right for you. Look for high quality fats and get the ones you need into your staple foods. You'll live longer *and* enjoy it more.

Chapter 12

The Skinny Girl Cooks

Cooking is the easy part.

Making the right choices, planning the right meals and maintaining the right attitude is the hard part. But, if you're this far, the hard part is over. The skinny girl cooks, but not without her cache of "secret" weapons. The first: a workable kitchen. I'm going to show you how to make putting together a delicious and healthy meal even easier – ok more attractive – than ordering a pizza every night or going through the drive through. How? A kitchen makeover.

The art of cooking will never go away. We have the technology to create little (or big) pills containing everything necessary for balanced nutrition. We could snack every day on "Monkey Chow," and still be in great health. But we love our food. It means too much to us. So we either cook, or have someone else cook for us. Maybe you don't have a personal chef or a spouse who aspires to the job. Well, then you have to set yourself up for success. That means having the ability to set up quickly, shop easily, and be able to store, prepare, cook, present and clean up the mess.

It also means we need recipes. Don't worry – they are *everywhere*. Magazines, newspapers, television, books, relatives, friends, the Internet, ancestors, chefs – good recipes are coming at you from all sides. There are people whose job it is to make up new recipes all day, every day. There are contests to come up with new recipes. You would need a Cray Supercomputer to calculate the recipes that can be made from just the typical foods on your grocery list. No wonder you are overwhelmed!!!

Taming the Recipe Monster

A long time ago, I read a Chinese cookbook by a chef who asked his readers point blank, "How many dishes do you need to be good at?" His answer was about ten – after that don't bother. His cooking instructions were so inscrutable and impossible to follow that I threw his book away. But I liked his main philosophy: you can't be an expert at everything, so don't even try.

Later, I read a book where the author asked her readers to look in their recipe clipping file and calculate how many decades it would take to try two of those new recipes a week. I had recipes stuffed into dozens of manila envelopes, and after I counted up to two centuries, I quit counting and decided to solve that problem.

Whether they know it or not, most people pick recipes in the same way they pick their staple food choices. They make the same things over and over from the foods they buy over and over. It can take a conscious effort to make some changes. Here's how:

Take your stack or drawer or cardboard box of recipes and sort them into little piles. You will find that most of the recipes fall into neat categories of versions of the same dish. I had 15 recipes for scallop brochettes and none for yellow squash. You can now organize them into a manageable form that is right for you, as well as add recipes that will complement the dishes you already make.

If you have managed to get this far in life without a huge stack of recipes, buy a cookbook and page through it. I like The Way to Cook by Julia Child. The hardback was $50, but I cook from it all the time. Julia Child has organized her book by cooking method, not the food itself, and I have done the same. For example, my stir-fries can be adapted to whatever meats or vegetables I have on hand, and still produce delicious results.

I purchased a little loose-leaf book with dividers for my loose recipes. The dividers separate nine different categories, including appetizers; dips, dressings and sauces; sushi and stir-fries; vegetables; soups and salads; kabobs and wraps; egg, rice and pasta main dishes; fruits and desserts; and beverages. Because this is *your* book, you can arrange it any way that suits you. I don't paste a recipe into my book before I try it. If I like it, it goes in the book; otherwise, it goes straight to the recycle bin.

When I looked at my recipes, I found repeats of nearly everything. Obviously, with 15 recipes, I like scallop brochettes. But how many variations do I really need? I looked at the common ingredients in each, picked the one I liked best for my recipe book, and *threw the rest away*. Now one recipe is at my fingertips; I just need to look in the cupboard. Do I have skewers, sauce, scallops and some vegetables? Dinner is just minutes away.

Look at your recipes *after* you have looked at the multi-vitamin you take every day. For example, my vitamin only supplies me with 20 percent of the magnesium and practically no potassium that I need, so I look to dietary sources of these. Fortunately, I like foods that are rich in magnesium, like green, leafy vegetables, nuts and whole grain breads so it's easy for me to pick foods that contain it. Unfortunately, I don't often eat bananas and oranges, which are rich sources of potassium, so I put a potassium and salt mixture in my saltshaker. Serious illnesses caused by clinical deficiencies of these minerals are rare, but I think my body can run low enough on them to cause changes in my habits – like low energy levels and potato chip cravings. These won't put me in the hospital, but they affect the *quality* of my life.

In the appendix you can compare your vitamins and your staple foods to see which nutrients you might be missing. I am not recommending you take a cupboard full of vitamins to make sure you get 100 percent of everything. Taking a multi-vitamin and eating a balanced diet of nutritious food you enjoy will take care of most of your needs. Look at the list of foods in the appendix and see which ones you could *add* to get the optimum nutrition you need to stay healthy and active. If you haven't done this yet, stop here and do it before we go on. You don't need to get out a calculator, but I figure if my vitamins and staple foods are giving me 80 to 120 percent of a nutrient, then that's enough to keep me going.

Now, when you go through your stacks, you will know exactly what kind of recipes you need to add to your repertoire and which you can just toss. "Palm Beach Salad," for example. It's a magnesium-rich main dish salad made with dark green lettuces, pecans and whole grain croutons. Delicious!

My recipe book has a permanent place on my counter in a plastic cookbook holder. I also have copied my favorite recipes from my cookbooks and pasted them into my counter book. I got a few strange looks when I carried a stack of cookbooks to the copy machine, but now I don't have to remember which recipe is from which book.

Now that you have your book, how do you eat healthy and tasty foods after dealing with customers, employees and co-workers all day? Not to mention the kids, the plumbing and the relatives. It won't be easy to get yourself set up, but once your kitchen makeover is complete, it will be a much easier task. Next, we are going to go through your kitchen twice – first to analyze your preparation areas, and the second to prepare a meal.

The Kitchen Makeover

When I walk into my kitchen, it's ready for me to get started. Getting your kitchen ready may take a little time, but once it's done, it only needs fine-tuning. Like anything else, you can be set up for success *or* failure.

When we are done, you will have a preparation area, cooking area, presentation area and leftover preparation area. They might be in the same 2-foot by 3-foot space, but each is separate and needs separate equipment.

I don't have to think about how I am going to pull a meal together, because I already *did* think about it, wrote it down and have a few things on hand to *actually do it well*. I am going to show you how to do this, too. This is where we start.

First things first. We are going to clean out all the cupboards. You probably needed to do it anyway, right? You don't have to empty everything out on the floor at once, but all of your drawers and cabinets are going to be rearranged to some extent.

We are going to start with the cabinet under the sink. Take everything out and have a good look.

Preparation Area

Never keep anything near the sink or in the kitchen that doesn't relate to food or washing dishes. So many people keep hazardous chemicals under their sinks for no good reason other than the fact that their parents did it. I keep dishwasher detergent and glass cleaner in a *lockable* cabinet with my pull-out garbage can next to my sink – that's all. Dishwashing liquid gets it's own pump dispenser on the counter so I can get to it with one hand. I have my scrubbies, sink stoppers and rubber gloves in a small pull-out rack that is camouflaged behind the fake drawer in front of the sink.

The garbage can is in a cabinet between the sink and the working counter space in the kitchen. It's convenient to toss out the waste from my projects, cooking or otherwise. The can slides in and out so it's there when I need it and out of sight if I don't. I don't have a trash compactor.

The cabinet door has a magnetic "tot lock" on it in case someone with small children visits. I flip the lock on my way to the door and that's one less problem I need to worry about. Children love to get into the lower cabinets. I have *nothing* they can't play with and a lot of peace of mind. Besides, you are going to need that space under the sink.

The real poisons, including alcohols, ammonias, lye, chlorine products, pesticides and everything else hazardous go out into my garage on a high shelf *away from the air conditioning intake*. The reason is this: those poisons are in solvents and many solvents are poisonous as well. The solvents evaporate into the air – your air and your family's air. That's what happened when you reach for the silver polish and found it all dried out: *the fumes went into your air*. That's why you want them as far away from you and your food as possible.

You especially don't want evaporated solvents being sucked into your air system and blown all through the house. The solvents ending "-ene" are especially deadly (xylene, toluene, benzene) and many of them can cause cancer. The cabinet under the sink is the *worst* spot for those items, and you don't use them in the kitchen, so why put them there in the first place?

Once you've moved those chemicals, clean the space under the sink until it is spotless. Look for any leaks in the plumbing and fix them immediately. Even a small drip will ruin the cabinet and attract bugs and mildew that cause allergies and aggravate asthma.

Put down cabinet liner and think about what you really want under there. I keep my cutting boards, colanders, veggie steamer, funnels and food strainers and baking accessories under my sink. I picked up an eight-inch high wire rack with five upright wires (making four sections) to keep my cutting boards and baking pans on their edges. I never have to move one item to get to another, which makes it very convenient. I can reach all of my cutting boards and colanders with one hand and don't need to take a step. They are right at the sink where I actually use them. This makes vegetable preparation a snap and *everybody* needs to eat more of those.

If you must have your dishwashing materials under the sink, put them in a shallow bin to contain spills and to keep from contaminating your other equipment. I keep a dish drainer inside one of my sinks to save on counter and cabinet space. It's flat white plastic with wavy slats that don't rust and is very unobtrusive. The slats are close enough together that I can use it as a colander when I'm in a hurry. I'm glad the kitchen equipment people are catching up with how we actually live today. Besides, I have a really small kitchen and every inch of space counts.

The sink area will be the start of your whole preparation area because almost every good recipe starts with washing *something*. Next to the sink (or as close as possible) you should keep your measurers, knives, mixing bowls and baking dishes. The measurers are not that important because, remember, you already measured out what a cup or a tablespoon looks like so you can pretty much do it by sight. Use that section of counter as your preparation area.

Empty the drawer under the counter next to the sink. Take it out and clean it really well. Think about how many sections you will need and get some dividers. You can buy plastic dividers at the discount store, but shoeboxes or their lids will do.

I have divided my utensils into sections by their use. I keep my clean dishcloths and towels in the section next to the sink. In another section, I have plastic measuring spoons and cups and two or three vegetable peelers – the kids love to help with measuring and peeling. (They're getting a math lesson, too, but don't tell them that.) Another section holds mixing spoons and stirrers. Still another has a small hand mixer and beaters. The last section has a selection of what I call "Weird Cutters That I Can't Live Without." This is where the pastry blender, pie cutter, egg and apple slicers and the potato masher stay. I also keep a selection of bamboo skewers for quick kabobs and brochettes.

I don't have a garlic press because I buy chopped garlic in two-pound jars. I used to buy those wonderful braided garlic ropes, where you pull off a head and lovingly peel and mash it with a bit of salt with a marble mortar and pestle to put in your homemade tomato sauce. Well, that was my life B.C. (before children). Right now that type of cooking is only a lovely dream. Now, I just scoop out the garlic I need and there's no clean up. There are no vampires around here and I spend *no* time using a toothpick to clean those teeny holes in the press!

I also have two hand held can openers: one on each side of my kitchen. Sometimes you open a can when you are preparing and sometimes you open a can when you are cooking. Because I want all of the things that I use in a section to *be* in each section, I sometimes buy multiples. Believe me, it is worth the extra $4.95.

Another word on can openers: I hate electric can openers. They are ugly and take up valuable counter space. You can't put them in the dishwasher (have you ever looked at the cutting edge of one?), they are useless in a power outage and they do nothing to strengthen your hands. Get handhelds – they are cheaper and superior to electrics in every way.

Knives, only three really good ones – a big chef's knife, a serrated knife and a paring knife – can either go in a wooden knife block on the counter or in a block in the drawer. They need to be protected because you paid a lot of money for them and they have important work to do. You don't want to be sharpening them every time you take them out.

In the cabinet under the drawer, I store preparation bowls and baking dishes. I have two sets of bowls, one glass and one plastic with lids. I usually mix my recipes in the glass bowls, but if something is going to be refrigerated for any length of time, I put it in the plastic. I keep the lids *under* the bowls so I don't have to go looking for them and only have three of each set. If you are using more than six bowls for any reason, I think you need to call a friend or the caterer.

I keep my Pyrex cooking pans and Pampered Chef Stoneware in the same cabinet. I can mix things up and then pour them into the appropriate baking dish. I switched from metal to Pyrex and Stoneware because metal can't go into the microwave. The Stoneware also is incredible for baking.

Take some time and measure a teaspoon of water into your coffee spoons and a tablespoon of water into your soupspoons. Look to see where the water reaches so you don't have to take out measuring spoons every time a recipe calls for a teaspoon of this or a tablespoon of that.

Cooking Area

The cooking area is the spot directly in front of and to the sides of the stove. Ideally, the stove has an oven with two racks and four burners. My microwave is right above the stove and under the ventilation fan. I use the microwave to cook foods that I would otherwise boil in water on top of the stove. I also use it for reheating leftovers.

You need a spot next to the stove for your cooking utensils. I have a cheap crockery container for a spatula, pasta fork, slotted spoon, ladle, steel whisk and a couple of bamboo spoons. Bamboo is superior to regular wooden ones because it doesn't leave splinters in your food.

I don't have a wall rack for utensils for two reasons. First, many of my utensils don't have holes in the handles and I like to look in only one place for the things I need. Second, I periodically take the crock and everything in it over to the dishwasher for a good scrubbing. Grease and dust accumulate in no time, and since I don't use all of them every week, I want to be able to wash them easily and have them ready when I need them.

For pots and pans, you need one or two saucepans with tight fitting lids, a sauté pan (it's shallow with sloping sides for quick cooking) and a large pot for boiling and stewing. I keep these in a drawer under my stove and in the cabinet on the right side.

Pots, pans and lids are a big investment like the knife. Get the best that you can afford. Mine are stainless steel with a copper sandwich in the bottom and fit perfectly in the dishwasher. The handles are attached with rivets, not screws, and are metal so they can go in the oven to stay warm, if necessary. They look as good as they did when I bought them 10 years ago. For everyday cooking, I use the stockpot, two saucepans and sauté pan. I only have four burners on my stove, so any extras are in storage. I don't have non-stick cookware because I always use a little fat when I cook. (Don't be jealous. You can do this, too.) I do have one non-stick coated sauté pan for making egg dishes though.

Above the cookware cabinet, I keep my herbs and spices and frequently used cooking condiments. I have seven kinds of vinegar and three kinds of cooking wine. I also have five kinds of oils and a bunch of different sauces like soy, Tabasco and Worcestershire. I also keep a few Pyrex custard cups in this cabinet so I can measure my ingredients into them beforehand and easily add them instead of flailing around at the last minute. Custard cups keep ingredients separated and are particularly convenient for Oriental cooking because it's done so quickly that you don't have time to measure once you start.

Everything else you need to prepare a good meal is up to you. I have a friend whose weekends are not complete unless she makes waffles, so she has a waffle iron. I gave mine away because I didn't want to clean it. I have a pressure cooker to cook things really quickly if I need to. Because they have new safety features, the previous dangers have been eliminated and they're great for making comfort foods. I also have a rice cooker with pre-measured markings on it for rice and water. I had to etch the markings myself, but it saves so much time because I prepare rice frequently. My wok, of course is very handy because I use it frequently, also. Take a look at the kitchen appliances you can't live without. If that Cuisinart has been collecting dust for the last six months, put it elsewhere. If a small appliance is not being used on a regular basis, you don't need it. Give it away or put it in the attic.

Learn to love the cheap hot pads and oven mitts from the grocery store. You really don't need the designer kind, and if you are going to be able to cook great things for yourself and your loved ones, you need to be able to do it with as little hassle as possible. You can't be worried about getting stains or burn marks on a $20 hot pad.

Also, everything I use on a daily basis goes in the dishwasher. If it will get ruined in the dishwasher, I have already ruined it and thrown it away. I don't need stuff that requires more care than I do.

Serving and Presentation Area

You should treat your food like you treat yourself: worthwhile and important. Don't go to any trouble to prepare something good and then eat it out of the pan over the sink. It's not fair to you or your food.

Your food should look good enough to eat. I knew a woman who told me she didn't care what it looked like or what it tasted like as long as she got it in front of her family. I was shocked. There is *power* in presentation. This woman was not using food as a source of strength and it showed in the rest of her life. She was miserable in every aspect. How can you live a complete life without enjoying your food?

I love looking at great table settings and appreciate those who can put them together with creativity and flair, but I am not one of them. I just buy dishes and table linens that are blue and white or some combination – no special shade – I use them all together. You could do something similar in any color you want. Your food will look it's best if the color is really vivid. "Vive" is French for "alive." Don't we all want to feel more alive?

Put an apple on a beige plate and right next to it put an apple on a blue and white plate. Which one "pops?" Stylists use the term "pop" to mean when something is so attractive that you have to pay attention. Well, if the apples and strawberries are popping in your refrigerator, aren't you going to pay attention to them instead of the chips? Bright reds or greens or yellows will bring out the personality of your fruits and vegetables and you'll go for them automatically – you won't be able to help yourself.

Use plates that are appropriate for the portion of food you are serving. I don't understand why some diet experts tell people to eat off smaller plates. If it's a ploy to get people to fool themselves, it sounds like a cruel joke to me. I have plates in a few different sizes because I like the look of different sized plates on a table.

Keep your plates and serving pieces next to the stove. Mine are in the upper and lower cabinets to the left of my stove. If you have a small family, you don't need a whole service for twelve in one cabinet. I split mine up to save room and get out the other half when I'm having a lot of people over.

Feel free to use your good dishes and nice napkins. Every day is a special occasion: don't shortchange yourself.

Leftover Preparation Area

Sometimes nobody asks for seconds during dinner, and I certainly can't eat all the food I cook, so I have a leftover station next to the refrigerator. In my small kitchen, the leftover station has to share the drawer with the cooking station. I keep plastic wraps, foils, zipper plastic bags and waxed paper in this drawer.

In the cabinet underneath, I have storage containers with lids in both plastic and microwave-safe china like Corningware or Pyrex. When I put foods away, it is convenient to divide them up into servings rather than putting the whole cooking pot into the 'fridge like a lot of people do. What you have now are your very own convenience foods. You can pop an appropriate portion into the microwave and dinner is done. What more could you ask for?

Throwing Food Away

If you want to control your weight the natural way, you must learn to throw food away. You can do all the tricks you want to do with leftovers, but once in a while you still have to throw good (or what was once good) food away. Do you feel guilty about that? Yes? Good. Instead of feeling useless guilt, use your guilt to help others who aren't as fortunate as you.

When you are finished with this massive reorganization, you will have your preparation area next to the sink. Your cooking area will be next to the stove. Your presentation area will be between the stove and your table and your leftover area will be next to the refrigerator.

Go through your cupboards and drawers, take out what you need, organize it for the job and get rid of the rest of it. I know this works because thin people are at home in each other's kitchens. There must be something to that. Take that leftover stuff and toss it, remake it or give it away, *but get it out of your life*. If you can do it with clothes, you can do it with your kitchen gear. You deserve to have everything in your kitchen working for you.

Food Storage

Now that your kitchen is clean and organized, you need to fill it with your food choices. Just as there is a system for working in the kitchen, there is one for storing foods properly to increase their lifespan.

Because my family was in the military, we went to "the commissary" for groceries. The base commissary was a dingy, crowded warehouse where people would buy food for months at a time. Everyone pushed two overflowing shopping carts and had to wait by the checkouts until carts came available. There would be arrows on the floor to point you in which direction to shop and heaven help you if you got out of line. We were like a line of camels, snaking our way through the aisles. One time, I got snagged in a jam that was so bad I had to laugh to keep from crying. And I almost did when the sergeant behind me barked: "Don't giggle! Just move!" as if I could just push the 50 people in front of me out of the way.

It was such a heinous shopping experience that most families set aside one day a month for the ordeal. Unfortunately, because the prices were so much lower than "on the economy," most families couldn't afford to shop anywhere else.

It was so awful that the day after my 16th birthday, my mother tossed me the keys to the family station wagon, handed me a blank check and told me to go to the commissary. The point of this story is that if you only grocery shop once a month, you get pretty darn good at food storage.

When you store foods, make a mental note of which foods will spoil first. Then eat those early in the week. Sometimes I have to stop myself from opening a can of green beans when I have fresh in the refrigerator. You can also buy fruits and vegetables in varying stages of ripeness and use them accordingly. Foods that spoil quickly include spinach, berries and cut melons. Cucumbers last for weeks until they're cut – then they'll spoil in a day or two unless they're pickled. Next in the perishables line are tomatoes, lettuces, grapes, summer squashes, peppers and "tree fruits" like pears and apples. Celery, carrots, winter squashes, onions and potatoes stay good for weeks. Cabbage lasts forever.

There also are all kinds of strange rules about what spoils if put together. For instance, onions give off fumes that spoil potatoes if they're stored together, and apples will speed the ripening of tomatoes if placed in the same bag. If you use all of these items frequently, like I do, you don't need to worry much about these rules.

I still freeze almost everything. I think I was 22 before I had a glass of milk that had never been frozen. Most meats, chicken, fish and shellfish will freeze well. Because you have already planned what you are eating during the week, it's a snap to take them out of the freezer and let them thaw in the fridge, where they will safely keep until you are ready to use them.

Bread products freeze well too. They will go stale in the refrigerator, but they thaw in no time when you are ready to use them. By buying fresh bakery bread and freezing it, you will be avoiding many of the trans-fats in factory bread without worry of it going stale or moldy.

If you want to make your own bread, it will keep in the freezer. A home-baker's love can't be duplicated. In European towns, the bread truck stops at the corner – like an ice cream truck – and the driver tosses out the unwrapped, fragrant loaves to the customers who gather. In the Bahamas, you can follow your nose to someone's home bakery and come away with a piece of heaven. While it's possible to find European style breads close by, I have never found decent Bahama Bread here in the states.

I also freeze milk, using half-gallon containers. I set one in the sink at night if I'm out of milk for tomorrow's breakfast. It is thawed by the time I am ready to use it – I just shake it *really well* to remix the cream before I open the container.

About the only thing that doesn't end up in my freezer is sour cream and cream cheese. Just about everything else winds up there eventually in a zipper bag of leftover chili and chicken soup.

When the onions, celery and carrots are getting a little past their prime, I make mirapoix. It's a French term for the chopped up vegetables that make the base of a whole lot of dishes, from soups to skillet dinners. I chop them up and freeze them in plastic bags. You simply break off a chunk and sauté. I don't use these for salads because freezing changes the texture, but it's not noticeable in cooked dishes.

I also have a great recipe for gazpacho that I make when my tomatoes and peppers are getting soft. I call it liquid salad and it's great as an appetizer or a meal itself.

Pre-Preparation

Remember that good knife I had you buy? Well, you are going to need it now. All those great fruits and vegetables and other foods need a little pre-preparation. A professional head chef has a person working for them called a prep chef. But just like many of us are our own housekeepers, we have to be our own prep chefs so everything is ready when the time crunch is on during mealtimes.

Go through your recipes and see if there is anything you can do ahead of time. You should have cut way back on the number of recipes you have. Unless cooking is your hobby, let's keep it simple. Sunday evenings are a good time for me to "take stock" and do some quick preparation for the coming week

For example, I like to drink mineral water with lime, so I keep a little dish with precut limes in the refrigerator. They last a few days and since they are right there, I have that instead of a canned soda.

I also pre-prepare Romaine lettuce (I like it better than Iceberg) by cutting off the bottom and pulling apart the leaves. Wash the lettuce thoroughly, let it dry and wrap it in a paper towel in a plastic bag in the refrigerator. It sounds like a lot of work, but it really saves time and aggravation in the long run because you can make that Chicken Caesar Salad or add lettuce to a sandwich because it's already washed and dried. Feel free to chop it with a knife. It's going to turn brown eventually no matter what you do with it, so if using a knife is the easiest way, go for it. Besides, do you really think the deli people hand shred their lettuce?

Don't forget that all important category of "grab and stuff." I keep a whole shelf in the refrigerator just for this purpose. I keep yogurt, fruits and anything else that fits my definition of convenience food. Wash the fruits you *want* to eat and put them in pretty bowls in the fridge. I like to keep strawberries in front of the chocolate so my husband sees them first.

Meal Preparation

Now that you are completely organized, you are ready to begin cooking. Follow this step-by-step process and the final result will be better and easier than you imagined. You can ask for help and everyone can pitch in, too.

If you are going to pull a meal together, you need to get some dishes dirty. First, run a sink (or basin if you don't have dual sinks) full of soapy water. As you work through the preparation process, toss your used utensils in the soapy water and you're halfway done with clean up already. You *know* the difference between a cook and a chef is who does the clean up. You need things working *for* you, not *against* you.

Many people soak their dishes after a meal and don't go back. Then, when it's time to prepare another meal, they are faced with a sink of dirty dishes and the next thing you know, the pizza guy is at the door again. Like I said before, I think pizza is nature's perfect food, but you can't eat the very same thing day after day and stay healthy.

When you have tossed your preparation utensils into the sink to soak, you or someone else, can wash them or put them in the dishwasher while you are waiting for your dinner to finish cooking. Half the mess is cleaned already.

Next, assemble your ingredients. The only thing worse than getting to the middle of the recipe and having to go to the market because you're out of eggs is having to start over with a new dish and less time. If you assemble your ingredients first, it's less you'll need to worry about.

Getting past the cleaning and assembly are my two biggest stumbling blocks to eating well. The rest is up to you and what you want to eat. Everything you need to turn out a great meal is now at your fingertips. You can get the cooking and presentation suggestions from the recipes. You have your ingredients and the pressure is off. It's a great feeling.

If I Didn't Mention This Already:

Get everyone involved. Yes, it's easier to do everything yourself, but by doing it the "easy" way, how much are you losing?

Many years ago, I woke up at 5 a.m. to peel potatoes for Christmas dinner. I was having the whole family over and I wanted everything to be perfect. I still remember the tears in my eyes as I watched the beautiful Christmas sunrise, all by myself, peeling those stinking potatoes! I swore at that moment I would never be so stupid again!

Now, it doesn't matter how mundane or special the occasion, I take time to delegate the jobs. Small children can wash green beans with you, instead of playing a video game. Older kids will feel like they're "a big help" in the kitchen. Teenagers will learn from your good examples when they need to get dinner on their own. You don't want to perpetuate the cycle of bad nutrition, do you?

Because I have pared down my recipe repertoire, I don't have to rack my brain to think of how to get some help. I even wrote a list called "Jobs for Kids" that I keep taped inside a cabinet for those times when I'm really under pressure. You can make up your own list when you are making your grocery list.

If you think that asking for help is a sign of weakness, stop it now. In the business world, it's called delegation and it's the basis for leveraging your efforts. The people who ask for help and get it are the ones in control.

Life is aggravating enough. I don't need the additional aggravation of trying to "do it all" myself, because I can't and don't want to do it all anyway. By asking for a little assistance, you can get in a little time with your family and make good meal preparation the high point of your day instead of the low.

Notes

Chapter 13

Recipes From
My Personal Collection

These recipes are not to be put on a 3-by-5-file card, but they are a way to cook and think about what your food is doing for you – not to you. These are jumping off points to inspire your own culinary creativity. If there is something you don't understand – ask a friend who might. Good cooks love to show off. You really need one basic cookbook to get familiar with the terms and the methods. Then, one day soon, you'll be showing off too, because food will be your strength, not your weakness.

I do like to roast a chicken or grill a steak now and then, but the old style of cooking (a meat and a potato every night) does not suit me. It's too time consuming, too expensive and doesn't provide me with what I need. While the popular alternative of hitting the drive through does save time and *seems* inexpensive, the trade off is poor nutrition and taste. I would gladly go out to dinner every night, but my schedule doesn't permit that anymore, so my choice is to cook well for my family and myself. To do that easily, I have spent years perfecting my techniques. What it all boils down to is this: I spend a lot of time washing vegetables and chopping them up, but I wouldn't have it any other way. One of my greatest pleasures is getting together with friends and family over a good meal we created ourselves. And I get to do that *almost* every day!

I only keep one thing in mind besides taste when I put a meal together – the Italian flag. I look for red, white and green on my plate. I don't count calories. I looked at my vitamins and saw I needed more greens to meet my mineral requirements. I also look at the fat content of my regular foods to see where I want my fats to come from. I don't do this every year – just when I have a lifestyle change, like a new job or home.

Take some time to experiment with the foods you love. Try to find more of them. The quality of your life will improve – *that* I can guarantee! My recipes are not so much distinct dishes, but methods of cooking that can be used with different foods: especially leftovers. If I were to make some nasty concoction from leftovers, I would just toss it out and start over. Fortunately, with the following techniques, that never seems to happen.

Beverages

Water

Water is the first and most important beverage. Of course no recipe is needed for this life-sustaining fluid, but you do need to think about where you are going to keep it so it's easy to get to when you need it. If you've been relying on the water fountain down the hall, you need more in your life. In Europe, the sanitation systems were built in the Middle Ages so people are used to getting their water from places other than the local plumbing. Drinking bottled water is the norm.

You don't need to buy expensive bottles yourself, but have a container nearby to take a sip when you need one. The first thing that goes on a construction truck in the morning is that huge yellow cooler of ice water. After that, they load the tools. At work, I have stored bottles of drinking water in everything from a Styrofoam cooler on the back floorboard of my car to a crystal champagne bucket on a silver tray on my fancy Queen Anne desk. Take a couple of the dollars you might feed into the vending machines and buy a six-pack of water. Stash it somewhere that is convenient for you, like a desk drawer or wherever you put your personal belongings at work. You need water like you need air to breath, and you need it to be close by or you will go without it.

Afternoon Cocktail

It's easy to add water and extra colors to your diet with beverages. Experiment a little. Mix any kind of fruit or vegetable juice with water, club soda, ginger ale, or tonic water. Garnish with a strawberry, lime, orange or lemon slices, or a celery or cucumber spear and serve it in a nice glass. Very refreshing!

Snacks & Appetizers

Think about where you usually are when you get hungry at different times during the day. What do you have on hand? Put some thought into how you can have good food available to you wherever you are. It might not be a bad idea to take your lunch to work now and then.

Think about the snacks you really like to eat. Then experiment with them and pair them with new foods for new tastes. These are the foods I like to have for snacks. It might seem like a lot of effort at first, but aren't you already putting a lot of effort into worrying about your weight? You might leave that bag of chips on the shelf for good.

Apples and Grapes

I haven't been able to bite directly into an apple since my adult teeth came in. It just feels funny. I bought one of those round fruit cutters that have eight sections surrounding a hole in the middle. It's a breeze to cut up an apple in one motion and there is no mess. I serve the sections with cheddar or Brie cheese, but they are delicious all by themselves. It takes about 20 seconds to slice one up to snack on as we are preparing our evening meal. It doesn't spoil dinner and can tide the little ones over until our meal is served.

If apples aren't appealing, try grapes. They are really juicy and already bite-sized, and are great as a snack on the run.

Fruit and Proscuitto or Cheese

Try wrapping thinly sliced pieces of ham around slices of honeydew melon, cantaloupe, apple or pear. Or do the same with Colby or Cheddar cheese.

Crudité

This is a fancy name for carrot and celery sticks. I don't care for them by themselves, but with a little salad dressing for dip, even the kids can't resist. I also use vegetables, like cucumber and lightly steamed broccoli and green beans. Cut up the broccoli and steam it for a minute or two in the microwave (or do it ahead of time) while you cut up the rest of the veggies. It will be ready in less than five minutes. I will do this instead of microwave popcorn once in a while for a tasty change.

Tapas and Bruschettas

These are baguette (French bread) slices with toppings. Make up your toppings ahead of time so they are ready when you are hungry. You also can toast the bread and then top it or top it first and put it under the broiler. Roasted red peppers, marinated mushrooms, marinated artichoke hearts, olive paste and cheese all make sophisticated snacks you can serve proudly. Go to the "olives and pickles" aisle in the grocery for ideas. You can keep a baguette in a bag the freezer and a selection of toppings in jars on hand so you will always have something good to eat – or a quick and elegant appetizer for unexpected guests.

Here is my favorite recipe for bruschetta. It's great by itself for an appetizer or at dinner as a side for pasta.

Bruschetta

1 or 2 fresh tomatoes, skinned and seeded and chopped
1 tablespoon fresh parsley, minced
1 tablespoon fresh basil, minced
1 teaspoon garlic, chopped
2 tablespoons extra virgin olive oil
1 tablespoon balsamic vinegar
Fresh pepper, salt

Mix all ingredients together. Brush French bread slices with some olive oil and broil or grill. Rub with garlic. Top the bread with the mixture just before eating. You can also add cheese, olives or mushrooms.

Sauces

The importance of sauces cannot be underestimated. What would Thanksgiving be without gravy? Or eggs benedict without the hollandaise? Sauces add flavor, color and texture to a meal that might otherwise be very bland. They can even be the basis for the meal itself if you have a lot of leftovers to deal with. If you can make two warm sauces and two cold sauces, even your closest friends will think you spent time in cooking class. Pick out a couple of these to try out on your family.

Warm Sauces

The first sauce to learn is Béchamel, the fancy French name for white sauce. It is the basis for hundreds of variations of fine meals, from the most humble to the most extravagant. Don't be intimidated when you see it called for in a recipe.

Basic White Sauce

White sauce and its variations is the basis for hundreds of meals.

2 tablespoons butter, melted
1 tablespoon flour
1 cup milk
Dash salt
Dash white pepper

Blend butter and flour together. Remove from heat and blend in milk. Cook and stir until thickened. Add seasonings and other ingredients as called for in your recipe. For a variation, try making the basic white sauce into a cheese sauce. Add ¾ cup grated cheese to white sauce and blend until melted. If the cheese is not pasteurized (like American), also add a half-teaspoon of dried mustard to emulsify and smooth it. You can use this to top broccoli and rice or add cooked macaroni and create great homemade mac and cheese.

The second sauce I make regularly is Velouté Sauce. We Americans refer to as gravy. This is the finishing touch to every roasted meal and a good many others as well. It is simply white sauce made with broth instead of milk. It's best when it's made in the cooking pan of your main dish, like roast beef, chicken or turkey, because the flavor essence of the meat collects in the bottom of the pan. However, any broth (canned or bullion) will do. It takes less than ten minutes.

Velouté Sauce

2 tablespoons butter, melted
1 tablespoon flour
1 cup broth
Dash salt
Dash white pepper

Blend butter and flour together. Remove from heat and blend in broth. Cook and stir until thickened. Add seasonings and other ingredients as called for in your recipe.

The last sauce I make regularly is a deglazing sauce, which means the sauce is made from the drippings in a cooking pan. It's the finishing touch to any meal.

Deglazing Sauce

Some recipes call for sautéing a piece of meat that has been coated in flour in a shallow pan. When the meat is removed, an easy sauce can be made from the flavor that remains. Just pour in some wine into the hot sauté pan. The wine, oil and flour emulsify to make a rich sauce. Add a tablespoon of butter and some other seasonings (parsley, mushrooms or onions) if you wish, simmer for a moment and pour over your main dish and a side.

For convenience sauces, I am partial to the Knorr-Swiss brands. They can all be microwaved for about five minutes in a Pyrex container. I find that some of their sauces can even taste better than my homemade versions. Imagine that!

Cold Sauces

Cold sauces are great accompaniments to meals and can make or break a dish.

Homemade Mayonnaise

This is the queen of cold sauces. A little goes a long way in any dish. I use a metal bowl that sets high in one of my saucepans as both a double boiler and a bowl for mixing the mayonnaise.

2 egg yolks
1 tablespoon Dijon mustard
2 teaspoons lemon juice, white wine or tarragon vinegar
Salt and freshly ground black pepper to taste
1 ½ cups peanut, canola or olive oil

Whisk the egg yolks, mustard, lemon juice, salt and pepper in a bowl set over simmering water until well combined and slightly thickened. Be careful not to scramble the eggs. Set aside to cool. Whisk a few drops of oil into the completely cooled egg mixture until it emulsifies. Continue steadily whisking small amounts of oil into the mixture until all of the oil is incorporated and you have a smooth sauce.
If the mayonnaise should "break," or de-emulsify, begin again with another tablespoon of mustard and incorporate the broken mayonnaise until you get a smooth sauce.

You can make many variations of the old favorite as well. My red pepper mayo makes a great spread for sandwiches and appetizers. Use it anytime you want a change of taste.

Red Pepper Mayonnaise

1 jar (7 oz.) roasted red peppers, diced
½ cup mayonnaise
1 teaspoon red wine vinegar
1 clove garlic, crushed

Combine all ingredients and mix well. Serve with deli-type sandwiches or as a dip for antipasto-type appetizers.

Green Sauce

This is a great cold sauce for any kind of dish or sandwich — especially cold roast beef.

1 large bunch of watercress or fresh spinach
½ cup mayonnaise
½ teaspoon lemon juice
¼ teaspoon salt
¼ teaspoon freshly ground pepper
1 ½ teaspoon chopped fresh tarragon or ½ teaspoons dried
½ cup plain yogurt
1 cup finely diced, peeled and seeded cucumber

Puree the first six ingredients in a blender or mix with a hand blender. Stir in the yogurt and the cucumber. Serve as a sandwich spread or salad dressing.

Another important cold sauce is a basic salad dressing. Some of the bottled types are great, but some of them are inferior, too. Next is one of my staple dressings.

Basic Salad Dressing

Mix ¼ cup olive oil with ¼ cup vinegar (any kind). Add ½ teaspoon mustard and mix well. Add garlic, grated fresh ginger, fresh or dried herbs and any other flavorings to your taste. You could also substitute the vinegar with fresh lemon or lime juice.

Fruits

Fruits are not only delicious, but some of them are loaded with enzymes that help digest foods, making the intestines work more efficiently. Which one's are they? There's a whole list on the side of the gelatin box. Pineapple, kiwi, papaya, fig and guava are fruits that you can't use in gelatin desserts because they won't allow the gelatin to set. This tells you instantly that there are enzymes at work in these fruits. Enzymes, such as Q10, speed up the cell chemistry that generates energy for every cell. Keep some of these on hand for snacks. Eating them will help your body digest other foods and get those good things into your blood stream faster. Gingerroot is also loaded with good things. I keep some in the freezer and grate off a little to use in cooking and dressings.

Herbs

Fresh herbs also are loaded with good things, as well as good taste. I buy parsley, basil and cilantro like other people buy houseplants – already grown in plastic pots. I slip the plastic pots into some pretty Italian ceramic pots that I bought specifically for the purpose – I don't even bother repotting the herbs. Parsley and basil can last for months in a sunny windowsill. Just snip off what you need. Cilantro won't last as long, but when the herbs have been used up, I just toss the pot of dirt into my garden and start over again. To use them in recipes, I put some in a Pyrex custard cup and snip them into little pieces with scissors. They are also handy garnishes for everything.

Every area has an "Herb Society." It was not so long ago that people went to their gardens for common remedies and these societies keep this body of knowledge alive. If you want to know more, you can call your county's Agricultural Extension Service and they can direct you to a meeting or two. You can also look for their recipe books and their plant sales. The books are often just typewritten sheets, copied over and over again, but they contain a treasure trove of wisdom.

Fruit Sauces

Here are two great fruit sauces that add a lot of color to your plate. You can make them with fresh pineapple, but mango and papaya will take you straight to the tropics.

Mango Salsa

2 ripe mangos, peeled and chopped
½ cup red pepper, diced
2 tablespoons purple onion, diced
2 tablespoons lime juice
1 tablespoon cilantro, chopped

Mix well and serve with fish, chicken or pork.

Papaya Salsa

2 ripe papayas, cubed
1 jalapeno pepper, diced (optional)
1 clove garlic
¼ cup red onion, diced
¼ cup cilantro, chopped
Lime zest
½ cup limejuice

Mix well and serve with fish or chicken or pork

Vegetables

Everyone needs more vegetables. There's no getting around that. They contain innumerable compounds that we are just beginning to understand. Some of these compounds are even as unstable as sparklers: they combine for an instant and then are gone, leaving their miraculous work behind. Our systems depend on getting the energy, nutrition and even the essential structure of plant foods to run their best. They were designed that way. You can swallow handfuls of vitamins and eat all the fortified foods you want, but if you don't have a least six ways to get fresh fruits and vegetables into your diet, you are headed for trouble.

Steaming Vegetables

Experiment with a vegetable steamer. I have a plastic one for the microwave and a metal one that fits in a saucepan. I add a cup of water or broth and steam any kind of vegetable, from 1 minute for spinach to 8 minutes for corn on the cob. You can top them with spray margarine, soy sauce or Parmesan cheese. Check your microwave's instruction manual and your basic cookbook for more ideas. There are a few recipes in the following section.

Basic Salad

I always start a salad with chopped lettuce, chopped tomatoes and shredded carrot. I used to hate carrots until a Cuban friend made me a salad with the carrots so finely shredded, I couldn't pick them out. After the first couple of bites, I realized the shredding released the best flavor and I have been shredding carrots into everything ever since.

Main Dish Salads

You can add anything you want to the basic salad and get great results. The produce department at your local market has shelves full of items that will enhance your "salad experience." Don't be afraid to use them. And if by some chance you make a mistake, toss it and start over. What have you lost? A couple of bucks? It's a small price to pay for good nutrition. Look at the next few recipes for inspiration.

Steak Salad

To the basic salad, add thinly sliced leftover steak, finely chopped onion and croutons. Drizzle with Italian dressing.

"Chinese" Chicken Salad

Bake some breaded chicken breast tenderloins according to package instructions. (Stoneware is great for this.) Cut in ½ inch wide strips. Serve over basic salad with chopped scallions, Chinese noodles and ginger dressing. Mandarin orange segments and crushed peanuts are good with this also. For those really in a hurry, pre-cooked chicken "tenders" are available.

Salad Nicoise

Arrange cut up romaine lettuce on a plate. Place some tuna (oil-packed tuna tastes best) in the center. Surround with quartered tomatoes, black olives, quartered hard-cooked eggs, cooked green beans, and slices of boiled and peeled new potatoes. Dress with garlic vinaigrette.

Palm Beach Salad

Arrange some chopped romaine lettuce on a plate or in a serving bowl. Top with drained and chopped oil-packed sun dried tomatoes and chopped apples. Sprinkle with crumbled Gorgonzola cheese, chopped pecans and whole grain bread croutons. Just before serving, drizzle on balsamic vinegar dressing.

Side Dishes

You've read two ways to prepare vegetables – leave them raw or steam them. But there are hundreds of ways to make great veggie dishes to accompany meat, poultry and fish. Here are some you may not have thought of.

Spaghetti Squash

Try using spaghetti squash instead of pasta with pasta sauce. They are yellow, football shaped gourds. Place it on the rack in the oven at 350° for one hour. Cut in half cross-wise, remove the seeds and allow to it drain in a colander or on paper towels before serving. To serve, take a big fork and pull out the flesh. It will come out in threads like spaghetti. The leftovers can be used instead of cabbage in a "coleslaw" salad with Italian dressing instead of mayonnaise.

Baked Sweet Potatoes

Sweet potatoes are one of the best foods you can eat. Wash and bake on the rack in the oven at 350° until soft, about a half hour to forty-five minutes. I don't wrap them in foil because if they aren't done when it's time to eat, I put them in the microwave for 5 to 7 minutes to finish. Serve with butter, salt and pepper.

Yellow Squash

In an ovenproof dish, cook two sliced yellow squash in a cup of chicken broth until tender. You can do this in the microwave or on top of the stove. Drain the chicken broth and top with grated cheese. Brown under the broiler until bubbly.

Steamed Asparagus

Wash asparagus and place in a gallon plastic zipper bag, along with some minced gingerroot and a piece of lemon zest and seal. Cook four minutes in the microwave (or until the bag pops) and top with a couple of tablespoons of vinaigrette dressing.

Spinach

Spinach deserves it's own section. I mentioned earlier how lucky I was that I had never tasted badly cooked spinach because my dad hated it. I still remember thinking, the first time I had a bite of spanakopita, Greek spinach pie, "How can people hate this stuff? It's delicious!" Here are some suggestions to get you started if you want to have more spinach in your life. You can use it in different ways for breakfast, lunch *and* dinner.

Spinach is delicate. Fresh spinach needs to be eaten within a few days of picking or it will go bad. Steam it in the microwave or sauté it in a little butter for a minute. As long as it still has the bright green color, it will be delicious. Overcooked spinach will turn bitter. If it turns dark, toss it out and start over. Frozen spinach is OK in certain dishes, but spinach from the produce stand is the best there is. There are thousands of great recipes you can use it in.

Breakfast

Sauté fresh spinach in a little butter or liquid margarine and serve it in egg dishes. I like to put some between an English muffin and a poached egg. It is also delicious in a Greek omelet with feta cheese.

My favorite spinach and egg breakfast is a French dish called Oeufs en Cocotte a la Florentine. It's one of the first "fancy" dishes a European child learns.

For each serving: Line an ovenproof bowl with a layer of cooked spinach. Break one or two eggs over the spinach. Set the bowls in a roasting pan filled with enough water to reach halfway up in a 350° oven. When the eggs are set, about 15 minutes, spoon thick cream (I use sour cream mixed with a little milk) on top and sprinkle with any kind of shredded cheese (I like Colby or Swiss). Brown for one minute under the broiler.

Lunch

One of my favorite salads is spinach – it makes a terrific lunch salad. Top it with chicken, salmon or beef if you like.

Spinach Salad

2 bunches of spinach, washed and torn
3 ounces slivered almonds
1 cup fresh mushroom, slices
3 hard-cooked eggs, sliced

Toss spinach, mushrooms and almonds together. Top with hard cooked egg. Drizzle on dressing (see below) before serving.

Dressing

3 tablespoons soy sauce
¾ cup brown sugar
1 small onion, grated
2 tablespoons Worcestershire sauce
1/3 cup catsup
½ teaspoon salt
¼ cup vinegar
1 cup oil, canola
3 teaspoons garlic

Mix all ingredients well.

This dressing also can be used as a marinade for chicken or beef. Make some extra or use the leftovers for brochettes later in the week.

Dinner

Here is a recipe I made up in desperation. It turned out to be pretty good and now you can have it also.

Red, White and Green Pasta Bake

½ lb shaped pasta (bowties, shells, etc. Tri-color pasta is pretty)
1 large bunch spinach, washed well
Butter or margarine
Tomato pasta sauce (homemade or from a jar)
Feta cheese (divided into two portions)
Grated Parmesan cheese

Cook pasta in a large amount of boiling water until al dente. Meanwhile, cook spinach in a small amount of margarine in an ovenproof casserole dish in the microwave for two minutes. Spread one portion of feta cheese on top of the spinach. When the pasta is cooked, drain and spread the pasta on top of the spinach and feta cheese. Pour some tomato sauce on top of the pasta. Spread the rest of the feta cheese and the Parmesan cheese on top of the pasta and sauce. Bake in a 350° oven for 30 minutes or until dish is bubbling and the cheese is lightly browned. Serve with garlic bread.

Soups

Soups are great either as a first course or as a meal. There are people who argue that all the nutrition in vegetables is released in cooking water. If that is true, then soup is the perfect dish to make. I try to make a homemade soup once a week and use the canned variety when I don't have time for anything else. Every good cookbook has a section on soups right in the front. There are tons of easy soup recipes. On the next page is a basic recipe you can add your own special touches to.

Basic Soup

3 cups of broth (chicken, beef or vegetable, canned, cubes or bases)
3 cups of cut-up vegetables (frozen, fresh or leftovers)
1 15-ounce can of diced stewed tomatoes
Salt, pepper, garlic and/or basil and oregano

Simmer for 30 minutes and serve.
You can also add canned beans, mushrooms, potatoes, pasta and cooked chicken.

Here is a recipe for when you need homemade chicken soup in a hurry. There is a reason it's called "Jewish Penicillin." I have even put the cooled, strained broth into a baby bottle or sippy cup for sick kids to drink – leaving out the cooking wine – of course.

Chicken Soup

3 cups water
1or 2 frozen boneless chicken breasts
2 ribs celery, julienne sliced (like matchsticks)
2 carrots julienne
½ small onion sliced thin or diced
1 teaspoon chicken bullion
Handful of noodles (any variety)
2 tablespoons vermouth, cooking wine or sherry (optional)

Bring the water to a boil. Drop in the frozen chicken breasts while you slice the vegetables. By the time you have finished chopping, the breasts should be thawed. Remove the chicken breasts. Skim the surface of the soup, if desired. Add the vegetables and bullion and turn the heat down to a simmer. Cut the chicken breasts into strips and return to the pot to finish cooking. Add the vermouth or cooking wine or sherry (if desired) and the noodles. Simmer on medium heat until the noodles are soft.

Gazpacho is liquid salad. I make it fairly often when my vegetables are getting a little soft. It keeps for days in the refrigerator and the flavors blend beautifully. You can serve it as a first course or as a light meal by itself. I actually had it served to me in a sculpted ice bowl at a fancy restaurant in Mexico, as we listened to a fabulous pianist in white tie and tails play a white grand piano. It was an amazing experience, but the following version tastes just as good on the patio on a hot day.

Gazpacho

1 ½ cups tomato or other vegetable juice
1 teaspoon beef bullion or 1 cube
1 tomato, chopped
¼ cup chopped unpeeled cucumber
2 tablespoons chopped green pepper
2 tablespoon wine vinegar
1 tablespoon canola oil
½ teaspoon salt
½ teaspoon Worcestershire sauce
1 or 2 drops hot sauce

Heat the tomato juice to boiling. Add the bullion cube; stir until it's dissolved. Remove the pot from heat and stir in the remaining ingredients. Chill several hours before serving.

Serve with croutons and a spoonful of sour cream. Ripe avocado is a great topping, too.

Breads

People have used grains as a staple in their diets since before recorded history. The four most common grains are wheat, corn, oats and rice. Bread and bread products are indispensable to a balanced diet, but too much of anything is not good. Most people get too much over-refined wheat and not enough of anything else. I get enough wheat, corn and rice without trying, so I make an effort to eat oat products because they don't automatically come my way. For this reason, I usually have an oat cereal for breakfast a few times a week.

Bread Machine

Everybody got one for a gift last year. Don't let it sit there and collect dust. Experiment with it and pick the recipe you like best if you want to add homemade bread to your repertoire. Look at your staple foods and add a recipe that will add to the variety of grains that you eat – like oats or whole grains. But don't try to make every kind of bread there is. That's what the baker is for.

Lastly, one day when you are up for a challenge, look for a recipe for piecrust dough or pâté brisee. With food processor, even inexperienced cooks can turn out a flaky crust and make a humble chicken potpie into a special treat.

The following recipes were mentioned in earlier chapters. Here they are so you don't have to do your own research.

Croutons

When your homemade bread goes stale, cut it into cubes and place them on a cookie sheet in a 325° oven. Stir occasionally and drizzle with olive oil or liquid margarine about halfway through, about 10 minutes. Continue stirring occasionally until the croutons are lightly browned, about 20 minutes total. They're perfect for all of those salads we talked about above. You can also crush them and keep them handy in the freezer to use a breadcrumb topping on casseroles.

Corn Bread

1 cup all purpose flour
¼ cup sugar
1 teaspoon baking powder
¾ teaspoon salt
1 cup yellow cornmeal
2 eggs
1 cup milk
¼ cup shortening

Sift the dry ingredients together. Add eggs, milk and shortening. Beat until smooth and pour into greased pan. (Stoneware is fabulous for this.) Bake at 425° for 20 to 25 minutes. Serve with the Hoppin' John recipe in the next section.

One Skillet Wonders

Most of my made from scratch meals are made in one skillet – less to clean up. They are generally made with foods cut into small pieces to release the flavor and cook quickly. A lot of the flavors blend so well; they actually taste better the second day. Most of these can be prepared in less than half an hour, but there are a couple that have to cook for at least two hours. Two hours is the minimum cooking time for less expensive cuts of meat to become tender. If you don't have that much time, fix something else. Or buy a crock-pot and let them simmer all day.

Browning Meats

It's important to leave a little space between pieces of meat when you brown them. If they are touching, the juices don't evaporate and the "browning" flavor that is so essential to the rest of the dish does not develop. This is important for beef stew, chili and the following chicken dish:

Pasta with Chicken and Asparagus

2 minced garlic cloves
¼ cup olive oil
½ pound boneless chicken strips
1 tablespoon sweet butter
¼ cup asparagus, chopped
¾ cup sun dried tomatoes in oil
1 tablespoon fresh basil, chopped fine
Pinch red pepper
¼ cup white wine
¾ cup chicken broth

½ pound cooked bow tie or other shaped pasta
Pepper to taste
Grated Parmesan cheese and pine nuts, if desired

Cut up the asparagus, sun-dried tomatoes, basil and chicken separately and set aside. In a large skillet over medium heat, brown the chicken and garlic in the oil; remove from skillet. In the same pan, add the butter and the asparagus; sauté until it is bright green. Add the chicken mixture, and stir in the remaining ingredients, except for the pasta, cheese and pine nuts. Cover and simmer for 20 minutes. Add the pasta and heat through. Serve with the grated cheese and pine nuts.

The following recipes are great on a blustery day. Some people say chili isn't chili if vegetables are in it. I add them because I like them, so you can call it whatever you want. The Hot Dish / Goulash is a quick version that can be ready in half an hour and the kids think they are getting macaroni and cheese, only better.

Basic Chili

1 pound ground or chopped meat
1 tablespoon vegetable oil
1 cup chopped onion
1 clove garlic
3 cups water
3 teaspoons beef soup base or bullion
1 large can tomatoes
1 large can tomato sauce
1 tablespoon chili powder
½ teaspoon ground cumin
1 bay leaf
1 teaspoon sugar

Brown the meat in a little oil. Add the onions and garlic and stir until cooked through. Add the rest of the ingredients and simmer for 30 minutes to two hours. You can also add kidney beans, white beans, and/or black beans, as well as an 11-ounce can of corn with liquid and 4 tablespoons chopped roasted red pepper. I also add cubed yellow or zucchini squash if I have it. Serve over rice with grated cheese and/or cornbread.

Hot Dish / Goulash

1 pound ground beef
1 bay leaf
1 small onion diced
1 large can tomatoes
1 can corn
Cooked macaroni
Shredded cheddar cheese

Brown the ground beef along with the bay leaf and onion. Add the canned tomatoes and corn. Let simmer for about 10 minutes. Add the cooked macaroni and heat through. Top with shredded cheddar cheese.

The next two recipes require a lengthy simmer, but are fairly easy to put together. I found the goulash recipe in Austria. When you go skiing in the Alps, you can take a break and warm up in these cute little huts on the sides of the mountains. There is always an old man in there tending a pot of this amazing stew to enjoy with hot cider. I don't know which is better, the skiing or the food. The beef stroganoff is what my mother always made for me on my birthday. It was also one of the things that attracted my husband to me. There's no fighting it: food really works!

Austrian Goulash

2 pounds beef chuck, cubed
¼ cup shortening
1 cup sliced onion
¾ cup ketchup
1 tablespoon brown sugar
2 tablespoons Worcestershire sauce
2 teaspoon salt
2 teaspoons paprika
1 teaspoon vinegar
1 clove garlic
½ teaspoon dry mustard
1½ cups water
2 tablespoons flour
¼ cup cold water

Brown the beef in hot shortening over medium heat. Add onion and cook and stir until onion is tender. Mix ketchup and seasonings; add to skillet and mix. Add 1½ cups water; cover and simmer two hours. Stir occasionally and add more water if the mixture gets too thick. Blend flour and ¼ cup cold water; stir into meat mixture. Simmer one minute. Serve over hot, cooked noodles with a dab of sour cream.

Beef Stroganoff

1 pound round steak, cut into strips
3 cups water
1 envelope dry onion soup mix
1 large can mushrooms
1 teaspoon bullion or 1 bullion cube
Hot cooked noodles

Brown the meat strips in batches. Add the water, onion soup mix, mushrooms and bullion. Let simmer two hours. Thicken sauce with 2 tablespoons cornstarch mixed in ¼ cup cold water. Serve over hot cooked noodles with a dab of sour cream and a side of cooked peas.

The next few recipes are lighter fish, pasta and rice dishes that are made with great tasting foods that do so much for you, you might want to make one or two every other week.

Tuna and Pasta

½ pound bow-tie pasta
¼ cup olive oil
2 tablespoons white wine vinegar
½ teaspoon salt
¼ teaspoon freshly ground pepper
½ teaspoon lemon juice
2 medium tomatoes, chopped
2 cans (6 oz. each) solid or chuck white tuna in oil, drained and broken into chunks
½ cup thinly sliced red onion
½ cup kalamata olives, pitted and coarsely chopped
¼ cup thinly sliced fresh basil leaves

Cook the pasta according to package instructions. Meanwhile, combine all the ingredients except the pasta in large serving bowl. Let stand 10 minutes to mix the flavors. Toss the drained, hot pasta with the tomato-tuna mixture. Serve immediately with rolls.

Mike's Fresh Fish

This is my husband's specialty. Mike catches the fish himself or gets it at the market and has them remove the "red" line.

Pour a little canola oil in a Pyrex baking dish. Place some firm fish fillets, (such as mahi mahi or grouper) in the pan and turn to coat. Shake on a little "Everglades Seasoning" or Paul Prudhomme's "Seafood Magic." Place the dish under the broiler for two to three minutes or until the fish begins to turn white.

Remove the dish from the broiler and turn the filets over. Season the other side and return to the broiler for an additional two to three minutes. The fish is done when it turns white all the way through and flakes easily with a fork.

Serve with yellow rice or black beans and rice. Sliced tomato and steamed spinach are great accompaniments as well as mango or papaya salsa.

This next dish is a New Year's tradition. It's so good and so easy; I make it frequently, even for guests.

Hoppin' John

Sauté some diced celery, carrots and onion in a tablespoon or two of butter. Add some diced ham (optional), a can of black-eyed peas, a bay leaf, ½ teaspoon of dried basil, and a dash of salt, black pepper and red pepper. Heat through. Serve over rice and garnish with shredded cheddar cheese, chopped tomato and thin-sliced green onion. Hot cornbread on the side is a great accompaniment.

This recipe is terrific fast food. Make the marinade, start the rice and then chop up some vegetables. Be sure to cook the denser vegetables, like carrots or bok choy first and add the lighter vegetables, like snow peas or spinach later in the cooking process.

Mi Sook's Stir Fry

For the marinade, mix together in glass bowl:
1 teaspoon garlic, minced
1 tablespoon ginger, grated
2 tablespoons soy sauce
1 tablespoon sesame oil
1 teaspoon sugar
Dash pepper

Cut beef, chicken or pork into thin strips about 3 inches long and place in the marinade for at least 30 minutes. Cut up assorted vegetables such as carrots, bok choy, broccoli, snow peas, green or red pepper strips, or whatever you have on hand. Canned water chestnuts and mushrooms also work well. Use the juice in place of the water for the sauce below if using them.

Heat a wok or high-sided sauté pan to high. Drain and reserve the marinade from the meat. Stir-fry the meat strips in 2 tablespoons peanut oil for two minutes. Remove from pan. Add a little more oil to the pan and stir-fry the vegetables for a minute or two. Add the meat back to the pan and heat through, stirring constantly.

Mix ½ cup water with 2 tablespoons cornstarch and add to the reserved marinade. Add the mixture to the pan and stir gently until the sauce thickens.

Serve over hot rice.

Cold Sesame Noodles

8 ounces pasta, such as linguini
2 tablespoons sesame oil

Sauce:
½ soy sauce
2 tablespoons tahini (sesame seed paste)
2 tablespoons sesame oil
2 tablespoons white vinegar
2 teaspoons minced gingerroot
2 cloves crushed garlic
2 tablespoons sliced scallions
2 tablespoons chopped roasted peanuts
Pepper to taste
Parsley, chopped
Snow peas, cut and lightly steamed

Cook pasta and drain. Toss with 2 tablespoons sesame oil. Chill. Just before serving, stir together the ingredients for the sauce and pour over noodles. Toss. Garnish with peanuts, parsley and snow pea pods.

This is also good when garnished with an egg sheet, tofu cubes, lightly steamed spinach and peeled, seeded and sliced cucumber.

Egg Sheet: Lightly beat one or two eggs. Heat 1 tablespoon of oil in a wok or similarly shaped pan. Add the egg, tilting the pan in all directions until the egg is cooked through in a thin layer. Slide the egg "sheet" onto a cutting board and cut into ½ inch wide strips.

Kabobs and Brochettes

Kabobs are those gigantic skewers of meat and vegetables that take up the whole grill. As much as I like them, I can't make them on the spur of the moment, even with good help. Brochettes are plate-sized kabobs that you can put together in a few minutes for a quick dinner. I usually serve about two per person. Nine-inch and six-inch bamboo skewers are available at the grocery. They should be soaked in water before using to prevent them from catching fire. Less expensive cuts of meat should be marinated a few hours beforehand, but chicken and seafood can be basted with marinade while cooking.

Beef Shish Kabob

1 to 2 pounds beef chuck
Marinade:
1 package dry onion soup mix
¼ cup brown sugar
¼ cup oil
½ cup ketchup
2 tablespoons mustard
2 tablespoons vinegar
1 ½ cups water

Cut beef chuck into 1-to-2-inch cubes. Combine the marinade ingredients in a saucepan. Simmer for two minutes and allow to cool. Marinate the beef chunks for a minimum of two hours and up to two days.
Thread onto skewers, alternating the meat with mushrooms, cherry tomatoes, peppers, pineapple, corn on the cob pieces, etc. Grill, basting with the remaining marinade. Serve with long grain and wild rice.

Scallop Brochettes

1 pound bay scallops
2 cups cherry tomatoes
2 cups small mushrooms, fresh
1 can pineapple chunks
1 green pepper, cut into one in squares
¼ cup cooking oil
¼ cup lemon juice
½ chopped parsley
¼ cup soy sauce (I like low sodium)
½ teaspoon salt
Pepper to taste

Place tomatoes, mushrooms, pineapple, green pepper, and scallops in a bowl. Combine oil, parsley, soy sauce, salt and pepper. Pour over scallop mixture and let stand for 30 minutes. Meanwhile, soak bamboo skewers in water.

Alternate scallops, mushroom, tomatoes and green peppers until the skewers are filled. Grill or broil about 4 minutes on moderately high heat. Baste with the reserved marinade Turn over and cook for two or three minutes more.

If you are in a hurry, you can substitute bottled marinade for the homemade. Serve with any type of rice.

Wraps

Tortillas are a kitchen wonder. Use flour ones to make wraps, which are really convenient because you can fix them ahead of time. Or use them for fajitas, so everybody can roll an endless variety of their own creation. You can find great recipes to make as a "new" meal or use up leftovers in a "new" incarnation.

This recipe came from a "Pampered Chef" Cookbook. It has everything I'm looking for when I prepare my meals. It's delicious, is made from a wide variety of fresh ingredients and only messes up one bowl. My experiences with their cookware, stoneware and accessories have been great. (www.PamperedChef.com)

Thai Tuna Wraps

2 tablespoons lime juice
½ cup mayonnaise, divided
1 tablespoon soy sauce
1 tablespoon sugar
3 cups cabbage, chopped
1 medium carrot, shredded
3 green onions, thinly sliced
2 tablespoons fresh cilantro, snipped
1 can (6 ounces) tuna, drained and flaked

6 8-inch tortillas
12-18 large spinach leaves
1 medium red pepper, cut into 24 strips.

In a large bowl, whisk together lime juice, 2 tablespoons of the mayonnaise, soy sauce and sugar. Lightly mix the cabbage, carrot, green onions, cilantro and tuna into the soy sauce mixture. Spread each tortilla with 1 tablespoon of mayonnaise and ½ cup tuna mixture. Cover with two or three spinach leaves and four red pepper strips. Roll up tightly and cut into 1-inch slices to serve as an appetizer or serve it cut in half on the diagonal as a sandwich. They can be made up to three hours ahead of time if wrapped in plastic and refrigerated.

Fajitas

½ cup Italian dressing
¼ cup limejuice
3 tablespoons soy sauce
¼ cup cilantro, chopped fine
3 green onions chopped fine
2 cloves garlic, minced
1 ½ pound beef flank steak, cut into thin strips
1 large onion sliced
2 or 3 red, green and yellow peppers, cored, seeded and sliced

12 tortillas
2 tomatoes chopped
Lettuce, guacamole, sour cream, cheddar cheese, salsa

Combine the first seven ingredients and marinate four hours or over night.

Remove the beef from the marinade, and add the onions and peppers to the same marinade and toss. In a large skillet, cook the meat in two batches so the strips are not touching and they brown evenly. Remove to a serving platter. Cook the vegetables in batches, and add to the platter. Discard the leftover marinade.

Heat tortillas according to package instructions and serve in separate dish.

Have each diner put a portion of meat and onion mixture in the center of a tortilla, add his or her own toppings and roll burrito fashion. Fold the bottom edge of the tortilla over the filling and roll up tight.

Beef and Cheese Burritos

1 pound ground beef
1 ¼ cups chunky salsa
½ pound pasteurized cheese
8 flour tortillas, warmed
Toppings:
Thinly sliced lettuce
Chopped tomato
Sliced ripe olive
Sour cream
Guacamole

In a large skillet, brown beef over medium-high heat. Pour off any drippings. Stir in salsa and cheese and heat until melted. To serve, give each diner a tortilla with about ½ cup of the beef mixture in the center. They can then add their choice of toppings. Fold the bottom edge over the filling and roll.

I also use leftover beans and rice or chili as the hot mixture.

BLT Wraps

4 slices bacon, cooked crisp and crumbled
3 tablespoons mayonnaise
½ cup sun dried tomatoes in oil, drained and chopped
Romaine lettuce leaves, center rib removed
4 flour tortillas

Combine mayonnaise and bacon. Spread each tortilla with a portion. Top each with some tomatoes and lettuce. Roll like a burrito. Chill until serving time.

Greek Wraps

1 pound button mushrooms, wiped clean with a damp paper towel
2 teaspoons olive oil
2 tablespoon lemon juice
1 16-ounce can of chickpeas, rinsed and drained
½ cup feta cheese, crumbled
2 medium tomatoes, sliced
Raita (recipe follows)
4 flour tortillas

Heat a grill or sauté pan to medium heat. Meanwhile, toss cleaned mushrooms with the olive oil and lemon juice in a bowl or a plastic bag.

Place the chickpeas, feta cheese and sliced tomatoes on a serving platter. Wrap the tortillas in foil.

Place the mushrooms on the grill and cook for two or three minutes, turning frequently. Heat the tortillas on a warm section of the grill.

Serve each diner a tortilla with some mushrooms in the center. They can then add their choice of topping, along with the raita, and wrap in burrito fashion.

Raita

1 scallion, finely chopped
1 cup chopped cucumber
1 clove minced garlic (about 1 teaspoon)
1 tablespoon lemon juice
1 teaspoon dried or 2 teaspoons fresh, chopped mint
1 ¼ cup plain yogurt

In a medium bowl, mix all ingredients.

The Summer Kitchen

Cooking outdoors is the great American summer pastime. Some of my neighbors have fabulous summer kitchens with professional quality grills, sinks and refrigerators built right into their patios. I think everyone should have a summer kitchen even if it's a $5 hibachi, a cooler and a hose in a bucket. Food just tastes better outside.

I use leftover grilled foods in the same way as any others – in salads or wraps. The grilled flavors give these dishes an unexpected and delicious twist.

Grilled Vegetables

I learned this recipe at a fancy party on Palm Beach one summer. Lightly grill some firm vegetables – summer squash and zucchini sliced in half lengthways are excellent. After they are cooked through, slice into chunks and drizzle with Italian dressing. Delicious!

Corn on the cob is great grilled too. Soak some fresh ears in the husk in water for about an hour (I don't even bother to take out the silk at this point, but some people do) then, grill over moderate coals for about 20 minutes or until the husks start burning. Be very careful when removing the cornhusks. They are very hot and very messy. To take off the husks, I wear a pair of (clean) suede work gloves and hold the ears down in a cardboard box or something similar to contain the mess. Serve with a little *real* butter and salt and pepper. Fantastic!

Two Great Leftover Recipes

These two recipes are great for the end of the week. With a few basic ingredients on hand, you never have to panic about putting a good meal together at the last minute. I use fresh ingredients when I have them, but it never hurts to have some frozen or canned items as a last minute back up. Just keep adding red and green ingredients.

Chicken Soup Pot Pie

1 can condensed cream of chicken soup
1 package frozen mixed vegetables, thawed
1 cup cubed cooked chicken
½ cup milk
1 egg
1 cup Bisquick baking mix

Preheat oven to 400°. In a 9-inch pie plate, mix the soup, vegetables and chicken.

Mix the milk, egg and Bisquick together. Pour over the chicken mixture. Bake 30 minutes or until golden. Serves four.

If you have time, this is even better if you mix your chicken and vegetable leftovers in your own béchamel sauce and bake it in a homemade piecrust.

Fried Rice

3 cups boiled rice
4 ounces shrimp
4 ounces ham or roast pork
8 ounces canned mushrooms
2 medium romaine leaves
1 green onion
2 tablespoons canola oil
2 beaten eggs
1/3 cup frozen peas
2 tablespoons chicken broth or soy sauce

Make an egg sheet as explained above and set the egg strips aside.

In a wok on high heat, stir-fry the shrimp, ham, mushrooms and peas together in the oil.

Add rice, green onion, and chicken broth. Stir-fry one minute.

Stir in egg strips. Cook 1 minute. Add romaine leaves cook one minute.

If all else fails, here is a good last resort meal that used to define the lowest point of home cooking. But it only proves that with a few special touches *anything* can be a family favorite. My sister, Janelle uses packaged puff pastry squares, but I use toast. You can also use canned tuna (drained) in place of the chipped beef.

Creamed Chipped Beef on Toast a lá Janelle

Sauté 2 tablespoons of diced onion in a little butter. Deglaze with ½ cup white wine. Add in 2 tablespoons of flour to make a roux. Cook and stir until the mixture is thick and bubbly. Season with a little dried tarragon and salt and pepper. Remove from heat briefly and stir in 2 cups of milk. Add chipped beef that has been soaked in boiling water, drained and chopped, as well as canned (drained) peas and mushrooms and heat through. Bake some puff pastry squares according to the package instructions. Serve the chipped beef over the pastry squares or toast.

One Final Note

Don't be overwhelmed by the recipes. They are only suggestions to add to your repertoire. I've had great results with all of them. If you look closely, they are made with the same ingredients, over and over again. If you did the kitchen makeover, everything you need should be right at your fingertips. But, don't make the mistake of becoming a short order cook for everyone. I don't take it personally if, for some reason, I get a "yuck" from someone. They are free to make *themselves* a peanut butter and jelly sandwich and enjoy it along with the rest of us. Most of the time though, when they are shown the bread cupboard, they just decide to join us.

Chapter 14

Living the Skinny Life

We know that diets don't work. Now, what do you have to lose by cleaning out your cupboards, getting your finances in order, eating breakfast every morning and playing with your kids? Nothing! These are the things I do every day and I haven't had an extra pound on me in 30 years. As far as I'm concerned, these are the ONLY things that work. It's the only program you can stick to day after day for the rest of your life and enjoy it, too.

Restricting what you eat cannot make you happier or smarter or more loveable. What is the mechanism? You'll be happier, smarter and more loveable when you don't isolate yourself and engage *all of you* in an interesting life.

The isolation begins the minute someone buys a "diet" product and puts her life on hold until she loses five pounds. Don't do this. If you are doing this – STOP IT RIGHT NOW!! The world needs you. It needs your strength. It needs your courage and it really needs your ability to overcome obstacles.

Living the "Skinny Life" is about enjoying life and having fun! And you can start it today. It is not about losing weight. It's about peace of mind and finding balance. It's really not a question of being thin or not. Too often, people go after the wrong prize. The goal should be creating balance in your life, and being happy with yourself while you pursue that balance.

It's about taking responsibility for yourself and asking, "What is my role in this?" Analyze your actions. Do you place blame on others for your problems? Do you see your job or your family or your other relationships as the root of all negativity in your life? If your relationships are truly causing you to do things that you know are wrong, change the relationship.

Everyone has problems. If you are not equipped to deal with your problems as a poor person or an overweight person, you still will not be able to cope with your problems as a rich person or a thin person. You may think that money or a new body will solve all of your problems, but it will just create a different set of problems. The key is to recognize *why* you have a problem in the first place and to get over your fear of confronting those problems. If you become an expert at *solving* problems, you will end up with the kinds of problems we all would love to have.

"Diets" don't work because you can't control your weight. You can't control your weight any more than you can control the growth of your hair. What you can control is what you feed yourself – physically, mentally, emotionally and spiritually. Every part of you needs nourishment. Give your body what it needs for nutrition and activity. It will pay you back by freeing your mind to love yourself. When you can love yourself, you can be genuinely generous and powerful.

When you are generous and powerful, you can use that power to help yourself or others make real changes in their lives. And when you can make a real change in someone's life, it makes you a person who *matters*.

The Lottery, Part II

I cannot stand it when perfectly rational people say they are going to do this or buy that when they win the lottery. If you are living in this time and space, you already have much more than any other human being who has come before you. More money will not help you. Besides, the things that people would do with lottery money are the same things people who haven't won the lottery do every day – buy a car, a house, finish their education. The same goes for losing weight.

When I hear people discuss what they plan to do once they lose weight or win the lottery, I think of medieval dragons, and the stories about their caves of treasure and beautiful women. But what are those dragons supposed to do with money and beautiful bodies? They can't use them. They are isolated in their caves, spending their whole existence accumulating money and bodies they will never use. Have you ever seen a dragon lying next to her boyfriend on a beach in Cancun?

If you put off your life until you have the treasure or the body you think you need for it, you are too late. The body you have here and now is the one that will help you achieve your hopes and dreams. How can it be otherwise?

The Multiplier Effect

Remember when we said, "All that math needs to put to a better use?" The better use is called the multiplier effect, or leverage. It is a chain reaction that works in ways, both positive and negative, in many aspects of our lives.

If you are sitting in a chair right now, grab the arms or the sides of the seat and try to lift it off the floor. It doesn't work. All the strength and willpower and wisdom you can muster won't help you lift that chair because you have no leverage. But, science museums often have exhibits of real cars hanging on the side of a big lever, with a rope hanging from the other side. Even five-year-olds can tug on the rope and lift the car that weighs a hundred times more than they do. That's leverage.

Leverage, or the multiplier effect, also works in the area of finance as "compound interest." Money is used to earn more money, and the total is used to earn even more. It works in education, social systems, or any area where people use "systems" to accomplish more than they could through sheer willpower and hard work.

You can leverage your habits into the life and body that you want. You can leverage concepts from all facets to set up a life that keeps you naturally thin. When your attitude is serving you, you can make better choices. A better choice will result in positive changes around you. These are *your* choices. Whatever you choose is going to be wrong to somebody, so it might as well be right for you.

Think through all of the consequences before you make those choices. Put your math ability to better use. Fill in the blanks in the following appendix and use what you learn to make changes that are right for you. Then go tutor a kid in math or science.

The factors you can ramp up to live "The Skinny Life" are Attitude, Activity, Breathing and Posture, Food Choices, Food Set Up, and Dealing with People. I see people making less than optimum choices in these areas all the time. But, no one wants advice from me because I *don't have a problem with weight and I wouldn't understand.*

If you think about it, it's not that hard at all.

From an emotional standpoint, the cycle goes like this: You do something that makes you feel good, either because you're being good to yourself or good to another. You're pleased with yourself for this deed and it shows. Later, you meet up with someone and he or she thinks, "This is a pleasant person, maybe we can do something fun together." You make plans, which means you'll be getting up and out. Now, you're using up energy and doing something that makes you feel good rather than sitting on the couch with a gallon of ice cream. And then the cycle continues.

From a physical standpoint, cycle goes like this: I take care of my back and my circulation system by choosing activities to keep them strong. Because my back is strong and straight, I can breathe properly, and because I breathe properly, I have a higher metabolism. Because my metabolism is higher, I can eat what I want. Again, by staying active, I take care of my circulation system. Because my circulation is healthy, I have more energy, and because I have more energy, I stave off depression and can enjoy my activities. And because I am doing fun activities, I am getting exercise and the cycle starts all over again.

I *don't* exercise to lose weight. I exercise to feel good. I exercise because I want my body to have the benefit of good nutrition and oxygen. Your activities, your exercise, should be something you enjoy so much that you look forward to it with anticipation – not agony. Luckily, hundreds of activities qualify as exercise – you just need to think about the activities you enjoy. I hope you have received a little inspiration to seek out activities *you* want to try.

You know you will get hungry a few times a day. Make your decisions ahead of time. Know what you will eat for your midmorning snack. If you don't plan, then what will happen when you get hungry? You'll take whatever is available. I know I need something to sip on, something to snack on and something to eat on the run.

Don't run on empty. What happens to an engine when it has low quality fuel or runs dry frequently? It is sluggish and it seizes up or stops running altogether. This is what happens to you if you skip breakfast or other crucial meals. Your body will compensate in ways you can't control. Give your body what it needs in the first place. You will be rewarded in ways you never thought possible.

The Disadvantages

There are several problems with being thin, however. One problem is garage sales. No one *ever* buys your clothes. In our town, once a year, we have a village-wide garage sale so everyone can trade their extra stuff to friends and neighbors. I had a nice display of items (remember, I used to display merchandise for a living), and all of my household items sold. At the end, as I was wheeling out a rack of clothes, one participant sarcastically commented on my obvious lack of success: "Oh, you poor thing, at least you tried." Well, they were all size two and four.

Because my weight doesn't fluctuate I can wear my clothes until they wear out and I often feel guilty about buying a new outfit when I still have nice ones in my closet. I sometimes accept invitations I might be tempted to skip because I have nothing to wear. I can't get away with that excuse. But, really it's a small price to pay.

Another downside to being thin is that people constantly try to feed me "diet" food. I refuse to eat that stuff. Sometimes, at social functions, another thin person and I will commiserate that we just don't like how it tastes. I don't eat diet anything. No diet sodas, no fake butter, no fake eggs, no fake bacon. I do not believe for a minute that over-processed foods are better for you than wise choices made thoughtfully and deliberately. I hate it when someone assumes I want a diet soda because I'm thin. The fake sugar gives me a headache. I really listen to my body when it comes to sugar substitutes. If I want a soda, I want a *soda*, not an inferior substitute. I do have one on occasion, but sodas aren't my first choice. I usually stick to water, lemonade, fruit and vegetable juices and milk.

This leads to yet another disadvantage – I don't use many coupons. It doesn't bother me that I don't spend Sunday mornings with scissors and color-coded envelopes. Years ago, I had a boyfriend whose mother thought I was a real spendthrift because I didn't use coupons. When she came to visit, she would shove the coupon section of the newspaper in my face and try to force me to start clipping. One day I told her, "If you can show me a coupon for a green pepper or a cucumber, I'll be happy to use it." Well, no such coupon exists. My usual food choices are predominantly unprocessed, so there is little or no profit that can be passed back to the consumer with coupons. Besides, if I won't buy it at full price, how could it be more appealing at 20 cents off? Certainly, I use coupons for paper, cleaning supplies, and canned foods, but over-processed foods are usually not on my list.

The Advantages

The advantages of living the skinny girl life far outweigh the disadvantages. If your size doesn't fluctuate, you only need one wardrobe. You can put together a workable wardrobe and actually have something to wear, whatever the occasion. Just like deciding beforehand as to what your food choices will be, you can decide beforehand as to what to have in your closet without having to panic because the outfit you picked out a few weeks ago for that big occasion still fits and looks fine, even terrific.

This is not the place to give wardrobe tips, but there is a system to having a workable wardrobe. And having a workable wardrobe can help you have a workable life. Think about where you go or where you would *like* to go and plan your wardrobe accordingly. For example, I like to go out dancing, and after a few years of marriage, I realized that we never went out dancing for fun anymore. I checked my husband's closet and realized that he didn't have any shoes that didn't have rubber bottoms. Well, going out dancing was never high on his list of priorities, but if I wanted to move it up, I had to take him out shoe shopping for the proper equipment. Sound familiar? I still can't get him to go out dancing very often, so I set up my own little disco in the garage so I can dance whenever I want.

For your wardrobe, buy clothes you need and use them. Seventy percent of life is just showing up dressed. You aren't going to go to the gym, nightclubs or the beach unless you have the proper attire. Think about what *you* want to do and set yourself up for it. At the clothing store, we would put together a stunning outfit for a customer and then have her skip it because she didn't have anywhere to wear it. We finally put together a list of places to tell customers where they could wear their fabulous new clothes. It was gratifying to tell a customer what to wear to a certain place and then see her there, later that week, scooping up compliments.

Consider the equipment you need to do what you want to do. I love my spiky heels, but I also have running shoes, garden clogs, tennis shoes, riding boots, mud and foul weather boots, hiking boots and boat and water shoes. This is in addition to my swim fins, ice skates, in-line skates and ski boots. If you men have only rubber-soled shoes or you women have only spike heels and flip-flops, you need to widen your radar screen and add some activities. Men need dancing shoes (the ladies love a man who dances) and women need something with *traction*.

Don't Hibernate

If you are going to have a life, you can't hibernate. You can't isolate yourself. Dieting is an insidious way for people to isolate themselves. Maybe you think you are making a connection with others by discussing your eating restrictions, but I think you are fooling yourself. Everything a body needs to be healthy and energetic is at the grocery store – today.

People need to do what is necessary to stay healthy and feel good. There are choices as to how people can approach life, so their activities are invigorating and sustaining, not wearing and tearing. Our bodies weren't designed to be sedentary. I try to do what I need to maintain my health and well-being, even if it's only five minutes a day. A lot of people depend on me, and I want to be in top mental and physical condition so I won't let them down. I reevaluate my food and activity inventories whenever I have a lifestyle change, such as a new job. It really only takes a few hours and it saves me a lot of aggravation.

I hope I have given you food for thought on how to evaluate your own life and make changes, if necessary. I've suggested things you can do, every day, for the rest of your life. If I can do this, you can too. Millions of thin people do these things, too.

Forward and Back

Your past has shaped this moment; this moment will shape your future. That one sentence is the source of my greatest hope and my deepest despair. It is what helps me to see things clearly and chart my life as I look at my past and my future. When you feel no motivation to change behaviors or habits, go back and read it again.

Everything you have done in your life, as well as those who have come before you, has brought you to this moment. What you do at this moment is shaping your future.

Concrete representations of your past and future are your "wish list" and "résumé." The wish list is a simple list of what you want in your life. Whenever I make a grocery list, whatever is on it eventually turns up in my cabinets. The same is true for other things in life. The simple act of putting something down on paper is the first step to making it real. If it only exists in my mind, it will never be "real." For me, the next steps just fall into place.

The résumé is a reminder of what I've accomplished. Some people call it a scrapbook, but I like to think of my life as more than scraps. Others keep a memory box and go through it once in a while. It helps you keep perspective on your life. Sometimes it's not what you have: It's what you have overcome. Find a way to be proud of who you are. So many people don't or can't appreciate the body they have. It was your very first gift in life and it will be your last. Take care of it.

The End

Notes

Appendix

I am not a nutritionist. I am a mom just trying to put good food on the family table day after day. I simply try to get the best use out of the information that is available to me. This is my method and I think it works well. I hope it works for you, too.

Food Guide Pyramid: http://www.nalusda.gov/fnic/Fpyr/pyramid.gif

Have a look at the food guide pyramid. Compare what you consider a "serving" to the pyramid's "serving size." You may find that what you consider an adequate serving is two or three times the recommended amount. You can adjust your portions accordingly and treat yourself to seconds if you are *really* still hungry.

Choosing a Multi-Vitamin:

If a vitamin has 80% or more of a nutrient, I don't need to make a special effort to make sure I have everything I need. I can get the rest from food. Some doctors say you can add 6 years to your life by taking a multi-vitamin every day.

Many commercial vitamins and cereals advertise "a whole day's worth of vitamins" yet still lack some essentials. If you don't get them from other sources, you will pay the price in a lack of energy and a less than optimal way of dealing with everyday stress.

In my general observation, common multi-vitamins come with varying amounts of vitamins, so you might want to look for one that has an abundance of nutrients commonly found in the foods you don't eat or don't care for. For examples, chromium is found in meats, cheeses, whole grains, eggs, fruits, and brewer's yeast. It is necessary for maintaining the normal metabolism of blood sugar. Some multi-vitamins have only 10% RDA of chromium, while others have 100%. If one is skipping carbs, doesn't care for fruit and eats no animal products, they could find themselves deficient and ought to pick one with a greater amount.

If you need to, take a magnifying glass with you when you shop for a vitamin. Subtract the percentage of each nutrient from 100. If the resulting number is more than 20, see the next section for sources. Look for food sources of these nutrients that you enjoy to *add* to the foods you eat on a regular basis.

My vitamin has:

A _____ % I still need _____.

C _____ % I still need _____.

D _____ % I still need _____.

E _____ % I still need _____.

K _____ % I still need _____.

B1 (Thiamin) _____ % I still need _____.

B2 (Riboflavin) _____ % I still need _____.

Niacin _____ % I still need _____.

Vitamin B6 _____ % I still need _____.

Folic Acid _____ % I still need _____.

B12 _____ % I still need _____.

Pantothenic Acid _____ % I still need _____.

Calcium _____ % I still need _____.

Iron _____ % I still need _____.

Phosphorus _____ % I still need _____.

Iodine _____ % I still need _____.

Biotin _____ % I still need _____.

Magnesium	_____ %	I still need _____.
Zinc	_____ %	I still need _____.
Manganese	_____ %	I still need _____.
Chromium	_____ %	I still need _____.
Molybdenum	_____ %	I still need _____.
Selenium	_____ %	I still need _____.
Chloride	_____ %	I still need _____.
Potassium	_____ %	I still need _____.

Sources

This is by no means a complete list of nutritional values. People have their own unique nutritional needs. It is intended to help you start to consciously choose the fuel that you and your family run on. You can get all of these foods by taking the outside circle at your grocery store. There is an overwhelming amount of nutritional information. If you feel you need additional help finding the right amount of vitamins and minerals for you, make an effort to find a source that you *trust*.

Years ago, liver served as everybody's multi-vitamin. It's a good source of many essential nutrients, but I don't care for it. Fortunately there are many great-tasting sources of everything your body needs to run. Look in the recipe section and you will find a dozen recipes that you can tailor to your own needs.

Don't try to get by without fiber. It gives your digestive system something to hold onto as it passes your food through your system. Fresh fruit and vegetables are high in fiber. Beans and legumes are great, too, as well as being filling and a good way to get complex carbohydrates and (when combined with a grain) protein. Seeds and nuts are also a good source of protein and essential fatty acids.

Vitamins A, K, E and D are fat soluble, which means that your body will store excess of these vitamins instead of disposing of them. This means that megadoses of these vitamins are toxic.

Vitamin A: cream, butter, egg yolk and liver.

Carotenes, from which Vitamin A is derived: yellow and green fruits and vegetables.

Vitamin C: citrus fruits, potatoes and their skins, tomatoes and green vegetables.

Vitamin D: fatty fish, eggs, liver, egg yolk and butter as well as fortified milk.

Vitamin E: vegetable oils, eggs and liver, spinach, olives and wheat germ.

Vitamin K: cabbage, cauliflower, spinach, egg yolk, and liver, as well as synthesis by bacteria in the gut.

Vitamin B1 (Thiamin): pork, whole wheat bread, whole grains and legumes as well as the outer layers of seeds.

Vitamin B2 (Riboflavin): milk, eggs, liver and green leafy vegetables.

Vitamin B3 (Niacin): unrefined grains and cereals, milk and lean meats.

Vitamin B6 (pyridoxine): wheat, corn, egg yolk, liver and lean meats.

Vitamin B12 (Cobalamine): whole milk, eggs, oysters, fresh shrimp, liver, pork and chicken.

Folic Acid: Green leafy vegetables, asparagus, lima beans, whole grain cereals, liver.

Biotin: present in almost all food, especially milk, egg yolk and liver

Pantothenic Acid: widely distributed, especially in eggs, yeast and liver.

Calcium: milk, cheeses, ice cream and other milk products.

Substitutes for milk: yogurt, tofu, broccoli, calcium-fortified orange juice.

Phosphorus: widely distributed in many foods.

Iron: dark green vegetables, eggs, soybeans, lean beef, fish, oysters and clams and baked potatoes.

Magnesium: whole grains, nuts, and green leafy vegetables.

Potassium: bananas, oranges, and orange juice.

Iodine: table salt.

Zinc: meat, eggs, liver, and seafood, especially oysters.

Manganese: whole grain products, nuts and seeds, avocado, dark green leafy, vegetables.

Chromium: meats, cheeses, whole grains, eggs, fruits, brewer's yeast.

Molybdenum: legumes, beans, lentils, peas, as well as whole grains.

Selenium: seafood, meat, cereals, grains.

Chloride: widely distributed in many foods.

Notes

Notes

Notes

On the Bookshelf:

The following books may not have been used as a direct reference in this book, but I have often referred to them for valuable information. They have not only help me to meet my goals and aspirations, but have helped me to deal with the stress of everyday living as well. They are in no particular order.

The Good Housekeeping Family Health and Medical Guide

Miss Manners' Guide to Excruciatingly Correct Behavior by Judith Martin

Home Comforts   The Art and Science of Keeping House by Cheryl Mendelson

Family Celebrations   Prayers, Poems and Toasts for Every Occasion by June Cotner

Lippincott's Illustrated Biochemistry by Pamela C. Champe and Richard A. Harvey

Caring for Your School-Age Child   Edward L. Schor, M.D., F.A.A.P., Editor-in-Chief

How Do I Look? The Complete Guide to Inner and Outer Beauty: From Cosmetics to Confidence by Gale Hayman

The Way to Cook by Julia Child

Notes

Notes

Order Form

Please send me _____ copies of Confessions of a Skinny Girl at $24.95 each. I am including $3.00 shipping for each book. Florida residents, please add 6% sales tax.

Send to: Balanced Life Publishing company
        PO Box 14944
        North Palm Beach, Fl 33408

By phone: 561-625-0250

E-mail: SkinnyBook@aol.com

Payment: _____Check payable to Balanced Life Publishing

_____ Visa _____ Mastercard _____ American Express

Card #_____ Exp. ____ Signature_____

Daytime Phone_____

Ship to:

Name_____

Address_____

City_____ State_____

Zip Code _____

Please allow 4 to 6 weeks for delivery.

Notes

Order Form

Please send me _____ copies of Confessions of a Skinny Girl
at $24.95 each. I am including $3.00 shipping for each book.
Florida residents, please add 6% sales tax.

Send to: Balanced Life Publishing company
       PO Box 14944
       North Palm Beach, Fl 33408

By phone: 561-625-0250

E-mail: SkinnyBook@aol.com

Payment: _____Check payable to Balanced Life Publishing

_____ Visa _____ Mastercard _____ American Express

Card #_____ Exp. ____ Signature_____

Daytime Phone_____

Ship to:

Name_____

Address_____

City_____ State_____

Zip Code _____

Please allow 4 to 6 weeks for delivery.